Living Life with Diabetes

Living Life with Diabetes

John Keeler

Edited by Barbara Millar

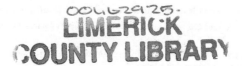
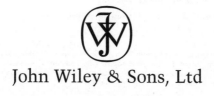
John Wiley & Sons, Ltd

Other Wiley Editorial Offices

John Wiley & Sons Inc., 111 River Street, Hoboken, NJ 07030, USA

Jossey-Bass, 989 Market Street, San Francisco, CA 94103-1741, USA

Wiley-VCH Verlag GmbH, Boschstr. 12, D-69469 Weinheim, Germany

John Wiley & Sons Australia Ltd, 33 Park Road, Milton, Queensland 4064, Australia

John Wiley & Sons (Asia) Pte Ltd, 2 Clementi Loop #02-01, Jin Xing Distripark, Singapore 129809

John Wiley & Sons Canada Ltd, 22 Worcester Road, Etobicoke, Ontario, Canada M9W 1L1

Wiley also publishes its books in a variety of electronic formats. Some content that appears in print may
not be available in electronic books.

Library of Congress Cataloging-in-Publication Data

Keeler, John, 1970–
    Living life with diabetes / by John Keeler ; edited by Barbara Millar.
        p. cm
    Includes index.
    ISBN 0-470-86913-5 (Paper : alk. paper)
    1. Keeler, John, 1970– – Health. 2. Diabetics – Ireland – Dublin – Biography.
    I. Title.
    RC660.4 .K44 2004
    362.196′462′0092 – dc22   2003023102

British Library Cataloguing in Publication Data

A catalogue record for this book is available from the British Library

ISBN 0-470-86913-5

Project management by Originator, Gt Yarmouth, Norfolk (typeset in 11½/13pt Imprint)
Printed and bound in Great Britain by TJ International Ltd, Padstow, Cornwall
This book is printed on acid-free paper responsibly manufactured from sustainable forestry in which at least
two trees are planted for each one used for paper production.

To everyone with diabetes, everywhere

Contents

About the author

Born in Dublin in 1970, John Keeler was diagnosed with diabetes on 15 May 1975.

He went to the BDA's (British Diabetes Association, now Diabetes UK) Youth Diabetic Weekend in 1996, and since then he became more involved with people with diabetes. He has facilitated many small groups both in Ireland and England, has been involved in the setting up of Ireland's young person's groups, counselled people with the condition, and has been a voluntary leader on many children's and teenager's diabetic camps.

John edited *Identity* (the magazine of the DFI [Diabetes Federation of Ireland]), now called *Diabetes Ireland*, from 2000 to 2001, and in 2001 he had an article published about his exploits at the European Masters Swimming Championships that year in Majorca, Spain, where he competed, published in *Diabetes Voice*, the magazine of the International Diabetes Federation (which is published in English, French and Spanish), where he competed.

In addition, he was a member of the record-breaking 'Four Peaks Challenge' team in 1997, has competed at the Irish judo championships, as well as many international club swim meets/ galas. John has, at various times, played soccer, Gaelic football, judo, qualified as a lifeguard, taught children how to swim, completed a distance-learning course in social sciences, gained a qualification in counselling, and plans to go into counselling/ psychology professionally, to work especially with people with diabetes.

Foreword

Diabetes mellitus is a growing problem. In the UK alone, 1.4 million people have diabetes and this figure is projected to grow to around 3 million by 2010.

This is the story of one person's life with Type 1 diabetes. John Keeler was diagnosed with the condition at the tender age of four years. He has no memory of life before diabetes. This book is his journey from that initial diagnosis through dealing with pain, fear and ignorance to his situation today, where he feels in control of his diabetes, rather than the condition controlling his life.

John is candid about the mistakes he has made along this journey. He is also forthright about where he feels he was failed by health care professionals, by work colleagues and by friends.

But this is not a self-pitying tale of adversity. Far from it. In describing his life with diabetes, John will inspire those with the condition to consider new challenges, and will inform those who do not have diabetes that a person with Type 1 diabetes is just like anyone else – they just happen to need insulin.

Understanding diabetes

Diabetes mellitus is a condition in which the amount of glucose (sugar) in the body is too high because the body cannot use it properly. Glucose comes from the digestion of starchy foods, such as bread, rice, potatoes, chapattis and yams, from sugar and sweet foods and from the liver, which makes glucose.

Insulin is a hormone produced by the pancreas which helps glucose to enter the cells, where it is used as fuel by the body. Insulin is the only hormone that can reduce blood glucose. When the insulin supply fails, the whole system goes out of balance.

Diabetes is a permanent change to a person's internal chemistry. The main symptoms of untreated diabetes are:

- increased thirst;
- going to the loo all the time, especially but not necessarily so at night;
- extreme tiredness;
- weight loss;
- genital itching or regular episodes of thrush;
- blurred vision.

The two main types of diabetes are:

- Type 1 – also known as insulin-dependent diabetes;
- Type 2 – also known as non-insulin-dependent diabetes.

John Keeler has Type 1 diabetes and this develops if the body is unable to produce any insulin. This type of diabetes usually appears before the age of 40 – John was just four years old – and is treated by insulin injections and diet. Regular exercise is also recommended.

The only way to determine whether you have diabetes is to have your doctor measure your blood sugar levels through a blood test.

It is an inescapable fact that people with diabetes have a higher chance of developing certain serious health problems including heart disease, stroke, high blood pressure, circulation problems, nerve damage and damage to the kidneys and eyes. The risk is particularly high for people with diabetes who are also very overweight, who smoke or who are not physically active.

You will greatly reduce your risk of developing any of these complications by controlling your blood glucose and blood pressure levels and by eating healthily and doing regular exercise.

In the last 10 to 20 years, the care for people with diabetes has improved dramatically. One of the most important developments has been improved methods of screening which will help your doctor to pick up any health problems at an early stage, so you can be treated more successfully. This is why having regular medical check-ups, at least annually, is so important.

Barbara Millar

Acknowledgements

My thanks to God and to Jesus His Son for everything; to my family, for all of their support; to Stacy, my wife – I love you; to Barbara Millar, who edited this work; to all involved at John Wiley & Sons Ltd; to John Grundy, for invaluable insights, advice and criticisms; to all at the DFI, both past and present; to everyone who was involved in the BDA/Diabetes UK's YD Weekends, especially my fellow facilitators, with whom I learned, trained and made some great friends; to the leaders and volunteers (both medics and non-medics) of our children's and teenager's diabetic camps for their help and great sense of fun; to the participants, for soakings, sleepless nights and joy-filled memories!; to all who went on the various young adult diabetic weekends in Fermanagh and Mayo; to the committee and families of the Sweetpea Kidz Club, whose work is immeasurably good, and to its helpers and volunteers; to all who pre-read this work and who gave me valuable feedback and encouragement; to all who have helped me on my journey; and to the reader – I hope this helps you in some way.

Introduction

Diabetes – what's that?

It's when my body does not produce insulin because my pancreas has packed up and will not work. I then have to inject insulin because I can no longer produce it.

So, having diabetes is just a case of replacing the insulin that your body no longer produces via injections ... that's easy! It just means you have to take an injection every day. Simple. End of story ...

I wish.

Diabetes not only has a physical effect on the lives of those of us who have the condition it also invokes many emotions which, in turn, also play a part in our well-being. The first reaction of people who have just been told they have diabetes is usually shock, fear and anxiety – all emotional responses, all strong and influential feelings. These feelings also have an effect on the way we begin to think about our future lives:

*What can't I eat? What **can** I eat? Can I drink? What do I do if I have one of those hypo [hypoglycaemic attack, see Glossary] things? What is a hypo anyway? What will happen if I forget to take my injection? Will*

I die? Will I go blind? If my blood sugar goes above 10, what damage will that cause? Will anyone understand? Will I be accepted?

Since you have been diagnosed, you have probably either considered or asked most of these questions. Diabetes, therefore, is not simply a physical condition, it also has a huge effect on our emotions and our way of thinking. It has a huge psychological impact that is largely ignored. But this does not mean that people with diabetes are in any way abnormal, or anything of the sort. It is quite normal to feel frightened, anxious, angry and often disconsolate about having diabetes. No one wants to have the condition, none of us can get rid of it and nothing we did brought it on – we did **not cause** it to happen to ourselves. But it is important to recognise our natural fears and anxieties about how we will cope with the disease.

People living with diabetes may also have a strong sense of isolation. It is very common to believe that no one knows what it is like to have diabetes – that you are the only one. I should know. I felt that way for over 20 years. And it is true, until you meet someone else who has it. Only a person with diabetes can possibly know what it is like to live with the condition, with all its tricks and subtleties. It can be so frustrating, especially when you feel the need to talk to someone about it.

There are people who will listen, but there is no one who really understands it. It is like a woman talking to me about what it feels like to be pregnant. I will just not be able to grasp it fully. I can try to understand, to sympathise and empathise, but, unless I have been pregnant, I just will not get it 100%. How could I? The pregnant woman will turn to someone who has been or is pregnant for comfort, advice and shared experiences. Why? Because that other person has gone through it. They really know what it is like. It is natural to turn to a person with first-hand experience of the situation. When you live with diabetes, you want to talk with other people who have had the same experiences. But, sometimes, that other person with diabetes can be so elusive.

Living with diabetes can also cause plain, downright fear. Fear is quite normal, but it also has negative effects on the way we live our lives. When, initially, we are diagnosed with diabetes, we are bombarded with information about what we can – and can't – eat, exercise, injection techniques, when and how often to check our blood sugar levels, what will happen to us if we so much as **look** at chocolate, or even cast an eye at that extra slice of toast, which suddenly takes on the allure of a gourmet meal.

Much of the information is negative, and it is often presented in an off-putting way. So, you stick rigidly to the new daily regime of blood test, injection, food allowance until, one day, BANG! That hypo hits you and leaves you reeling. You feel the symptoms – the shakes, the tingling in the tongue, the weakness, the heat, the sweats and the panic, which can be worse than the rest of the feelings put together.

You might manage to get through the hypo – either on your own, or with help – but the experience terrifies you so much that you promise yourself that you will never have to go through it again. You begin to eat – sweets, cakes, biscuits, chocolate – even if the blood tests show your level to be 7 or 8 mmol/l – just to ward off that potential hypo you fear so much. In some cases you may give up a favourite activity, something that was once your passion, but which you force to become a distant memory.

Horrible decisions to make – unnecessary even – but perfectly understandable. I have felt all of the above – and more, as I'm sure you have too. But it does **not** have to be like this. You can take the power to control your diabetes instead of letting it control you.

This book is my story. The story of how I, John Keeler, became diabetic and the effects this condition has had on me and on my life. Many of the opinions in the book are mine and may not be shared by others, including you. But that's the thing about people – we are different in so many ways – some obvious, some less so.

This is my story.

He couldn't want so much water

In May 1975 my younger brother and I caught measles. I was four years old, Peter was three. We were put into bed – the same bed – until we recovered. Eventually, our spots disappeared, but even after they had gone I did not make the expected recovery. I was always thirsty and constantly asked my mum and dad for glasses of water. One night, when my grandparents were staying with us, I went downstairs for a glass of water to quench my raging thirst. Ten minutes later, I went down again. And then again. And again.

Finally, one of the grown-ups said, in a mixture of exasperation and concern: 'He couldn't possibly want so much water!' But I did need to drink a lot, and it was decided that I should be taken to the local GP. He simply bent down, smelled my breath, and pronounced: 'Diabetes!' We were then sent to the Harcourt Street Hospital in Dublin.

I can still recall the corridor of the hospital on that night – 15 May 1975. It must have been quite late, as it was dark. I remember sitting on a chair, apart and away from the doctors, nurses and my parents, who were all on the other side of the corridor, huddled in what seemed to me to be a conspiratorial manner. The medical staff were informing my parents about the need to admit me to hospital to investigate

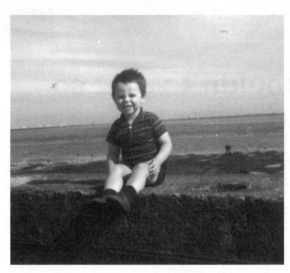

Figure 1   John – two years before diagnosis, July 1973.

this *diabetes* thing – or at least what they knew about it then –
and about how long I would have to stay.

From where I was sitting, though, it all looked rather
sinister. Being only four years old and being told that I would
have to stay in hospital while my parents went home only
confirmed my suspicions that they were all out to get me!

I spent six long weeks in hospital, such was the lack of
knowledge and information about the condition at the time.
Sometimes, I was allowed out for the day, but, when
I thought I had finally escaped, I soon discovered that I was
expected to return the very same night. One morning, as I was
dressing myself in anticipation of being collected, a nurse asked
me why I was getting dressed. When I said that I was going
home, she answered: 'No, you're not.' This completely
terrified me – I honestly thought I would have to spend the
rest of my life in that hospital.

It was decided that I should be getting more exercise, so
I was told to run up and down the stairs. This confused me –
why couldn't I use the lift like everyone else? And what was
I going up and down the stairs for anyway? My dad also took
me out to St Stephen's Green, in Dublin city centre, on
occasions. There he would time me as I ran round the park.

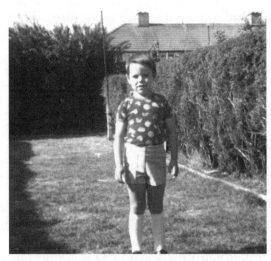

Figure 2 John – two months after diagnosis, July 1975.

After I had left the hospital, I recall one of the nurses who had cared for me there coming to our house to pay me a visit. I still have a vivid image of a bright, sunny day and that nurse – whose name and face I can sadly no longer remember – playing football with us in our back garden. This was a very generous and selfless thing to do, I now realise, but I am glad I still remember that special day. This sort of gesture, by a member of the medical profession, can really make a difference. The personal touch, the aftercare, for which overtime is neither sought nor paid, is very valuable.

I am from a fairly Catholic family background and I believe very much in God. It is something I have inherited from my parents, to my delight. A couple of years after I was diagnosed, it was suggested that I was taken to Lourdes in the south of France. In fact, I remember my grandfather saying to my parents: 'Send him to Lourdes.' I was horrified. At seven years of age, this sounded as though I was being banished. I had still not come to terms with being taken into hospital, away from my parents, when I was four – now this!

Lourdes is a town in the French Pyrenees which is visited by millions of people because of its reputation for healing people through their faith. In February 1858 Our Lady appeared to Bernadette Soubirous, a young peasant girl, on several occasions and told the young girl to search in a nearby grotto, where she would find a spring.

News quickly spread that drinking water from this spring would provide a miracle cure for a variety of illnesses. Since then, the grotto has been visited by people from every walk of life, who come in search of a cure. Parish pilgrimages from Ireland have been regular events, and my dad and I went on one of these in October 1978.

While we were there I bathed three times in the freezing cold waters. After five days we returned home. The visit to Lourdes made a lasting impression on me, and it definitely brought me closer to God, which has made my life much more complete. I was not, however, cured.

I had a problem with bedwetting as a child, which I now know to be the result of having raised blood sugars at bedtime. I had no glucometer (see Glossary) to check my levels – this was in the 1970s – so a great deal of my lifestyle and treatment was down to guesswork. I now know that one of the side effects of raised blood sugar is an increase in the amount of urine to be passed. But back then I simply thought I was weird. My younger brothers had well grown out of the stage of wetting the bed, while I seemed to be getting left behind. I carried a lot of needless guilt and shame about this, negative emotions caused by diabetes. These were to influence my life as a teenager, and, even now as an adult, some of those feelings still persist.

When I returned to school in September 1975, I explained to a classmate that I had been in hospital for six weeks during the holidays. Naturally, he asked what was wrong with me. 'I am a diabetic,' I told him. 'Oh,' was his response, 'so you're allergic to sugar.' I suppose that this other boy, who was only the same age as me and I am aware I should make allowances for five-year-olds, must have heard this response from someone older. Obviously, his informant did not have much of an idea about diabetes. This was my first encounter with some of the myths and misconceptions about diabetes, which I would have to challenge throughout my life.

My school bag was always packed with sandwiches and a

plastic container of milk, which I had to drink at breaktimes. But, many times, I would open my bag to find that the milk had spilt from the container and soaked my books and papers, all dripping wet with stale, smelly milk. This was a nightmare then, though I can laugh about it now. Another memory that springs to mind is of realising, one day, that I had forgotten my 'life-saving' sandwiches. I was a very timid child, and, when I began to appreciate the enormity of the problem, I began to cry so much I could not stop.

One of my classmates went to get my brother, to see whether he would be able to stop me crying, and I vividly recall Peter galloping toward me, all the time stuffing his own sandwiches into his mouth. This memory now prompts a wry smile. It reminds me of the terror, the absolute dread that I felt so often during my childhood. When I knew that someone had gone to get Peter, I felt relieved. I knew that he would give me his sandwiches. But when I saw him actually eating those sandwiches, I was paralysed with fear. I really thought that I might die. I would never, ever, want anyone to experience the feelings I had that day. Even as I write this, I am reliving that fear, all because I had done something as trivial as forgetting my sandwiches.

Eventually, a teacher saw me and asked what was going on. I sniffled my way through an explanation and was then given some of the milk and sandwiches supplied to the school each day. I was saved. But I never again want to experience the fear I felt that day. As a child it affected me greatly. It helped to sap my self-confidence for years. The feelings of dread also really knocked the stuffing out of me for a long time. That was something I feel I did not deserve.

Sometimes, my usual class teacher was absent. I hated this happening as it involved the class being broken up into groups and sent into different classes until it was time to go home. I had to try to explain to the new teacher that I had to eat at certain times, even sometimes during lessons, which was usually frowned on. Every time this situation arose, my heart thumped as I tried to convince the teacher that I was not an attention seeker; it was just the safest way for me to get through the day.

In the 1970s the world seemed to be mystified by diabetes and so was I. At the end of a whining and invariably unsuccessful attempt at explaining my predicament, I usually ended up blurting out: 'Diabetic!' It almost always ended with me in tears, which shocked the teacher and amused my classmates. I hated those times.

One day, I was walking to school with my precious container of milk in my bag. Slightly late, I was running across the road and, as I ran, the container of milk fell out and rolled into the road. Having had it drilled into me how important to my well-being drinking milk was, I turned, ran into the road and grabbed it. It never entered my mind to look left and right. My only thought was 'I have to get my milk. It is vital to my health.' As I was bending down in the middle of the road, I was almost knocked down by a van coming round the corner. He hit the brakes just in time and I grabbed the milk container, turned and ran away. Ironically, it was a milk delivery van that had almost hit me!

For the first few years, the way I knew whether my sugars were up or down was through urine testing. This required me to wee in a pot, in order for me to extract five drops of urine, which I would add to a test tube along with ten drops of water, then put in an acidic tablet, which would dissolve in a fizz. There was a scale to measure how much sugar was in my urine: navy blue meant there was none; dark green meant there was a 'trace' of sugar; three progressively lighter shades of green indicated more sugar was present; and bright orange meant there was a lot of sugar present.

Every day I would come home from school and do one of these tests, and every time I would eagerly anticipate the concoction in the test tube turning navy blue. I was usually disappointed, as it often went bright orange. Sometimes, however, it was a shade of green and, very occasionally, it did go navy. I loved this. It could mean an ice cream or a bar of chocolate for me – heaven!

Because I was diagnosed at a time when knowledge of diabetes was not as advanced as it is nowadays and information was not as readily available, I was encouraged to try the 'diabetic foods' of the time. Diabetic jam, diabetic

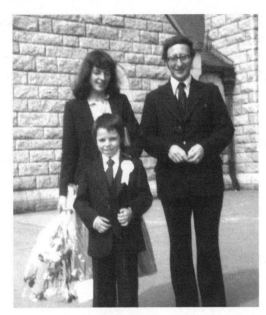

Figure 3   John – first Holy Communion, May 1978.

biscuits and diabetic chocolate were great ideas, except for one thing – they tasted awful, except perhaps for the biscuits, as they seemed to have been made without any taste whatsoever!

When a pot of diabetic jam was brought home I would eagerly anticipate a major treat – bread and jam. I would butter the bread, open the pot, scoop out as much jam as I could get onto the knife, spread it richly all over the bread, drop the knife and hungrily take a bite. All the time I would be thinking about how good this was going to be. I am having bread and JAM! I would begin to chew, my taste buds tingling in anticipation of the treat to come. Then the 'flavour' would hit – and it was indescribable. Argghh!! Take it away! The lid would be firmly replaced on the pot and it would be hidden at the very back of the kitchen cupboard.

Ages later, this experience having been long forgotten, something in the cupboard would be moved, revealing the hidden pot of jam and I would decide to try it again. The lid was opened and then I would need to step back, holding it at arm's length and trying to decide whether it was worth scraping the old man's beard off the top of the remains of the jam. It was truly gruesome.

Not only were the diabetic jams devoid of flavour, they were also a waste of money, as they never were finished and were always thrown out. Nowadays, with our knowledge, we can eat ordinary jam on bread, without it causing too many problems. There is also a much better quality of sugar-free foods now available. But, a few years ago people with diabetes were stuck with largely tasteless foods. How times have changed.

Why me?

When I went into secondary school, the history teacher gave us the creation of a family tree as a homework project. We also had to present it to the rest of the class. When it was my turn, as part of my own history, I mentioned that I had had diabetes since I was four. Then came a question that stumped me. 'What is diabetes?' asked a classmate.

I was really taken aback as I really did not know what it was. As far as I was concerned, diabetes meant injecting myself daily, watching what I had to eat, avoiding chocolates and sweets – unless I was playing football or swimming – and, on occasions, feeling 'funny', 'dizzy' or 'hungry', which were my words for being low or hypo. I could not answer this question.

I was rescued by the teacher who said it would take too long to explain. This experience should have been the trigger for me to find out about diabetes for myself, but I didn't do much about educating myself on the subject until several years later. Maybe it was a form of rejection of the condition, an unconscious decision – who knows? All I knew then was what I had been told at diagnosis at the age of four. 'Inject "this". Do not eat "that", unless you are playing football.' I carried these instructions in my head for years. How did I survive? I will never know how I did not end up in hospital with diabetic ketoacidosis (DKA).

DKA occurs when there is no insulin present in the system – either because it has not been injected or, when the insulin that had been in the system has been completely used up. This results in ketones – acids – appearing in the blood and urine. The usual signs of DKA are extreme nausea, vomiting, stomach ache, drowsiness and a sickly sweet smell on the breath. DKA feels really, really bad and can also be extremely dangerous.

Insulin must be given intravenously in cases of DKA. Also, because of the increased amount of acid in the system, blood flow decreases, preventing oxygen being carried to the brain. The more acids or ketones formed, the greater the risk. The person can end up becoming ketotic.

Of course, not everyone who has a raised blood sugar level will become ketotic. However, we should all be aware of what can happen if our bloods get out of hand (e.g., after going on a binge or not bothering with our injections). It is much easier to prevent this from happening in the first place than trying to deal with it.

We all have blood sugar readings of 15 mmol/l and above every now and then, and this will not do too much harm. But **do not** let the blood sugar level continue to creep up. Keep an eye on your blood sugar level, take into account what you have been or will be doing and do your best to prevent DKA – it is horrible and very dangerous.

When insulin is finally introduced into a ketotic vein, large quantities of it are required, as the insulin must fight extremely hard against all the acid present in order to diminish the ketones. This in turn will allow the blood to flow back through the veins.

Looking back, I can remember times when I was hit by DKA first thing in the morning, especially through my teens. I would have eaten way too much, far more than was recommended, the previous night and, when I woke the next morning, I would not even be able to stand, the feeling would be so overpowering. I would try to get up, collapse and wonder what on earth had gone wrong. I'd take my injection and try to force myself to eat – because I did not know I was ketotic and did not understand about insulin adjustment back then – but, usually, I would not manage even a mouthful and would simply fall back into bed and doze off and on. I always felt better lying down. A couple of hours later, I would feel well enough to get up and then I'd go back to living in ignorance about what had happened.

Adolescence is a weird and unpredictable enough time in anyone's life – and I was no exception. I also had this diabetes albatross hanging round my neck and, as well as encountering the usual teenage mood swings, I also had to contend with other emotions that seemed unique to me. Later I was to discover that the emotions are quite common among people with diabetes.

For example, how do you feel when you have eaten chocolate or cakes, sweets, ice cream, biscuits – the *nice-tasting stuff*? Better? Full? Thirsty, due to a rise in your blood sugars? What about **guilty**?

I have often eaten chocolate simply because I wanted it. But then I have felt as if I have done something terribly wrong and I feel as if I should apologise for having wanted to taste it. Sounds crazy, I know. But sometimes that guilt feeling is there, which is why I think the worse ingredient in chocolate is not sugar, or fat or any of that. It is guilt.

Guilt is not necessarily a logical feeling, but it can be a very strong one. A lot of people with diabetes have told me that they too have felt guilty for having diabetes and imagine that, if they had done something differently, then they would not have 'caught' it. This is just not true. No one who has Type 1 diabetes could have stopped themselves from getting it. Eating too much sugar does not turn you into a diabetic. It just happens. No matter what you did or what your parents, siblings, friends, anyone, did or did not do would have prevented it from happening. Having diabetes **is not your fault**. If we knew how to prevent it, someone would have won a Nobel Prize by now!

There are various theories around which give differing opinions of the causes of diabetes. One theory suggests that it needs a 'trigger' to become visible and that those of us who have it were born with diabetes, but it did not show itself until something activated it. I caught measles when I was four years

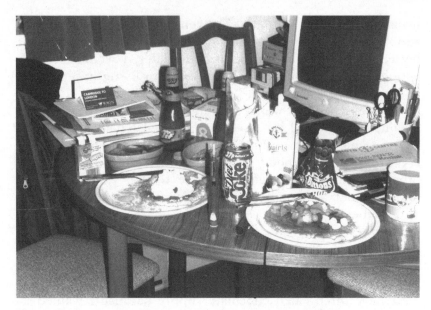

Figure 4   Should I or shouldn't I?

old, at the same time as my younger brother. He did not get diabetes, but I did. I did feel as if I had been singled out and, as we played football as children, often I would have to disappear mid-game to eat, which did not make me the most popular player on the pitch. This led to feelings of guilt which would gnaw away at me for years. Guilt even made me feel ashamed at times, especially if I went 'low'. Why?

When I was hypo, my behaviour was often strange and other people had to take care of me. I felt as if I was an imposition on everyone around me and that, if it were not for my going 'low', everyone else would be much happier. Everything felt as if it was my fault. If I did not have diabetes, everyone else would be much better off. My having the condition meant others had to suffer.

Guilt is a feeling that seems to be experienced by many people with diabetes. It is illogical to feel guilty – having diabetes is not our fault – but the feeling can be so acute, so real. Perhaps it has something to do with believing that hypos are a loss of control, a control which we are constantly not only told that we 'should' have but which we 'should' also be very good at. Therefore, hypos = loss of control = failure, leading to guilt.

I don't think I was too rebellious as a teenager, but any rebelliousness manifested itself through my battles with diabetes. I hated hearing that I could not have chocolate and I actually ate tons of the stuff during my teens, sometimes through need, often out of desire and from time to time just out of plain greed.

The feeling of *needing* to eat chocolate is interesting. Often, our blood sugar level will drop to a point where chocolate is actually permitted, even required, from a physical point of view – to prevent a hypo. Sometimes, if you have been very well disciplined over the previous few weeks and have not given into the desire to put some of that delicious substance into your mouth, you simply want to savour its tempting sweetness. You see everyone around you indulging themselves and think: why not? You go ahead and eat some. OK, your blood sugar level no doubt will rise. It might even increase quite rapidly. But you *feel* so much better for having tasted the chocolate. In a totally different way, it has actually done you the world of good, even if it does mean you having a raised blood sugar. So what? The odd raised blood sugar every now and then will not kill you **BUT** you must make sure that it is only now and then – it can be a hard habit to break.

There are ways of being able to enjoy chocolate from time to time, such as doing exercise or taking more insulin. If you want an opinion on the different tastes and qualities of the various chocolate bars on offer, as a person with diabetes – we are the real experts!

At the age of 14, I went on to a twice-daily injection regime, one in the morning, one at evening mealtime. One evening some of us were out playing football. It wasn't long after my evening meal and I was on this occasion playing in goal. The ball was down the other end of the pitch when I felt an itch on my arm, and scratched it. As I did, it suddenly hit me that I had not had my evening insulin. I still wasn't used to having to do it in the evening and injecting into my arm was also a new step for me.

I started to panic – but quickly realised that this was pointless. I was only a short way from my house. I had to leave the field, mid-game, went home, took my insulin and got back into the game. There were no adverse effects – except perhaps our team being a goalie short for a couple of minutes – and it helped me to remember that I was now on two injections a day.

I was on a mixture of *Actrapid* and *Monotard* (see Glossary) insulins back then. Monotard was a long-lasting insulin, while Actrapid, as the name conveys, was fast-acting. I was advised to inject Actrapid 20–30 minutes before a meal. I was concerned, however, that this would not always be practical. What if I took my injection and then something happened before my mealtime? What if I injected and then had to leave the building because of an alarm (this actually happened to me at work a few years later)? What if I was in a restaurant and there was an unforeseen delay in the meal being served?

My concerns meant that I generally gave myself the injection just before my meal, not giving it a chance to get into my system. As a result, I was not getting the most out of it. Instead of maintaining a steady blood glucose level with the Actrapid beginning to work as I began to eat, the Actrapid was being taken just before I ate, with the result that my blood sugar levels were already raised before the insulin began to work. The Actrapid had to catch up with the soaring blood sugar level in order to bring it back down, instead of preventing it from rising in the first place, which was the whole idea of having the injection half an hour before the meal!

Of course, this caused problems of raised blood sugar levels and consternation from the medics who could not understand why my HbA1c (see Glossary) results were so elevated. With hindsight, I can see that I must have had numerous hypers (hyperglycaemic attack, see Glossary) without realising it. I also had lots of hypos without knowing why. Every Friday, just before lunch, I would without fail have a horrible low, or hypo. It would hit me just before 1 p.m. I would become tired, hungry, agitated, sweaty, sometimes completely exhausted, and I would crave the ringing of the lunchtime bell almost as much as I craved the energy-giving food. I knew that I was going to feel bad, but I did not have a clue how to prevent it from happening. The hypos often left me with whoppers of headaches, which lingered on for a long time. Later on, from talking with other people with diabetes, I learned the splitting headaches were the side effects of massive hypos.

I joined a swimming club and swam regularly, every Thursday and Friday. During the school holidays we would also be taken on day trips by the swimming club. A favourite spot was called Claralara, in the Wicklow Mountains. This was a big fun park, with a lake, rafts, boats, swings, rope bridges. Once, when we were about to leave the park, we were waiting on the bus for the remaining stragglers to arrive. This coincided with my evening injection time.

As pen injections were not then routinely available, I was still using the old plastic syringes to draw up the insulin from its glass container. As we sat there, on the bus, I took the opportunity to prepare and inject my insulin. As I started to give myself the injection, I spotted another coach, full of foreign students, all of whom were gazing at me with jaws dropped. I found this attention extremely embarrassing and off-putting, but at that moment the bus pulled away and I was saved from further mortification. For a long time, however, I shied away from injecting myself in front of people whom I did not know.

Those students who had seen me injecting insulin had looked horrified, some even disgusted, at what I was doing. I had not been able to explain what I was up to and realised they probably thought I was on drugs. This experience affected me for a long time afterwards.

I also suffered with a horrible, diabetes-related ailment called *balanitis*. Balanitis is terrible. Thank goodness I only had it a couple of times, although I did not then know what it was, nor what caused it. When you have balanitis, the top of the penis becomes sore and the foreskin becomes thickened (called *phimosis*), due to infection with yeasts that, it seems, thrive on the high concentration of sugar in this particular region. In women there is itching or soreness around the vagina, which is called *pruris vulvae*. Urination becomes painful and distressing. I was afraid to go to the toilet because of the pain. Too much sugar, however, makes those of us with diabetes need to urinate more frequently – the perfect nightmare combination! If the urine is kept clear of sugar through better control, when the blood sugar level drops the balanitis/pruris vulvae will clear up.

I wish I had known that, when it happened to me. I was in my teens when it first occurred, a time when I was too self-conscious to tell anyone about it. I was terrified. I was also disgusted with myself as I thought ... well, to be honest, I did not know what to think. No one had ever warned me about balanitis and phimosis and it caused me fear, anguish, worry and shame – all of which could have been avoided if someone had explained to me what these conditions were, how they might occur and how they could be treated. Even if you have a good relationship with your medical team of advisers, this is still an awkward and often embarrassing subject to talk about.

If these conditions have happened to you, you are **NOT** a freak. The conditions are treatable and, with good control over sugar in the urine and helped by anti-yeast cream, will clear up. If these conditions do occur, tell your doctor, if you can. If you cannot, make sure you get your sugar levels down, being careful to avoid hypos.

I have also been through a phase that I imagine most of us with diabetes will have experienced – hating the condition. Injections are daily – 7 days a week, 52 weeks a year and, in most cases, there are more than one a day. That can be tough. There are also blood tests, if you do them, which again can cause pain and discomfort. There is the threat of hypos, the fear of having your blood sugar rise too much, the constant pressure to **get it right**. No wonder people hate having diabetes. You may also have to explain it wherever you go and will often be frustrated by the general lack of understanding, both of how diabetes affects us and how we feel about having it. It is an awful situation to have to face, but there it is and there it remains, and there is not a whole lot we can do about it.

I began to wonder: why did I get diabetes? Why me? 'Why me?' is a question I am sure we have all asked. Not getting any satisfactory answer made me angry, and I would often express my anger verbally. However, the reaction to this anger was to be told that I was feeling low and then I was almost force-fed!

Anger can be a symptom of hypoglycaemia but it can also be a reaction to injustice, physical pain, lack of under-standing ... take your pick from any number of things, including having diabetes. It is so annoying to have feelings brushed aside with a patronising comment such as: 'Oh, you must be low' and then be handed a bottle or a biscuit or a bar of chocolate and told: 'Take this and you will soon be OK.' I was OK to begin with!

Not every angry person with diabetes is hypoglycaemic. I have often been extremely 'low' and laughing my head off. Also my anger tends to increase – justifiably, I feel – when the points I am trying to make are not taken seriously, sometimes not even acknowledged. So, forget about a calm-me-down, fix-me-up chocolate bar. LISTEN TO ME!

Another aspect of hypos can be a loss of control. Once, I remember throwing a cup across the room during a hypo, narrowly missing my brother's head. I knew what I was going to do. I also knew that I should not do it, but I still could not prevent myself from doing it. What if I had hit him? Imagine the shame, the guilt, the anguish. Thankfully, I did not, and someone came in to rescue us both. That's another thing – once in a hypo, you usually have to rely on someone else to help you get out of it. What if there is no one there? Think about that, think of the possible consequences and you may then understand the fear people with diabetes often feel.

We are not to blame for having diabetes. It is not our fault. It is NOT our fault. **IT IS NOT OUR FAULT!** It is **OK** to be angry and upset about having diabetes. I think it is better to express true feelings so that, hopefully, they can be dealt with. If we continue to contain our anger, it becomes buried, often deep within us, until we contain so much that it overflows and we EXPLODE with frustration. Yes, diabetes is tough and yes, it is for ever, unless a cure can be found, but such is life for us. We may have had no choice in getting diabetes, but we can choose to live with it. Help is there for those who want and need it – although it is not always easy to find.

Tips and hints

Stress

Stress can be a very real problem for people with diabetes. The diagnosis of the condition or the diagnosis of complications are stressful for many people and can also be stressful for close relatives.

For people with diabetes, stress can affect blood sugars. Under stress, the body produces hormones, such as adrenaline. These hormones cause the body to release stored glucose and fat for the extra energy required to deal with the stress, but they can only be used provided the body has enough insulin.

It is this sudden extra production of glucose in people with diabetes that causes blood sugars to rise. This can be made worse by the way many people react to stress – by overeating or taking less exercise because of a lack of energy. Exercise, however, will not only help to make blood sugar, it is also recommended as a way of helping people to cope with stress.

General tips for coping with stress include:

- avoid nicotine, too much coffee, alcohol or tranquillisers;
- work off stress – physical activity is a terrific outlet;
- don't put off relaxing;
- get enough sleep to recharge your batteries;
- learn to accept what you cannot change;
- manage your time better and learn to delegate;
- know when you are tired and do something about it;
- if you become sick, don't carry on as if you aren't;
- plan ahead by saying 'no' – you may prevent too much pressure building up in future;
- maintain a sense of humour!

3

When did you last hear an orange say 'Ouch!'?

I remember a story I was told of a boy who had been diagnosed as having diabetes. After he had been discharged from hospital, his mother noticed that at mealtimes her son would flail his arms around for a few seconds in a violent, windmill fashion, rather like Pete Townshend during his days with The Who. Knowing that he had gone through an ordeal, his mother initially did not question his strange actions. Finally, however, after weeks and weeks of the same, arm-flailing mealtime ritual, curiosity overcame her and she asked him why he was waving his arms about. He replied: 'Well, the doctor told me I should rotate the injection site ...'

When I was diagnosed, I was taught to inject myself in my thigh. As I entered my teens, I was then shown how to inject into my arms. I even became able to do this left-handed, which is pretty difficult for a right-handed person. Next, I was shown how to inject into my backside and became proficient with both hands, but I was 20 years old before I finally did my first stomach injection. (Admit it, you thought I was going to say before I could sit down again, didn't you?). So, various parts of my body have endured over 25,000 injections, by my reckoning. But one thing is common to all of these injection sites – they can become quite sore.

I am not a bodybuilder with a six-pack stomach, but I am not fat around the gut either. My fleshy area is from my hips to a few centimetres from my navel. The first time I carried out a stomach injection, it seemed an easy enough task. All I had to do was choose a spot and inject into a very accessible site. But, as I prepared to perform this task, I hesitated, I winced, my eyes were shut tight at one stage, until I eventually jabbed in the offensive weapon. IT HURT! It was an injection, after all.

Even now, several years later, I almost always momentarily hesitate before injecting into my stomach. Often, I emit an involuntary, but loud, hiss as I insert the needle. People who see me doing this usually ask if it hurts. I say yes, it often does hurt. At other times it is not so bad. What I hate, however, is being told, dismissively: 'That shouldn't hurt you.' How would they know? Is what they are really saying: 'That wouldn't hurt me'? It is very easy to be brave when you don't have to go through it. It is an easy enough procedure and yes, it is only a small jab, but most people do not have to contemplate sticking a sharp object into their body simply in order to eat.

It is OK to admit that injections can hurt. What is the point in saying that they don't, if they do? Sure, a lot of the time it is relatively painless, but it can also be quite sore and painful.

I do not worry about my injections. I know that they must be done and I have sometimes had to give myself six injections in a day, mainly due to my voracious appetite. But, for the split second it takes to puncture the skin, it does play on my mind. Once it is done, though, that is it – it's done, it's over. I know those people who are educating newly diagnosed people with diabetes point out that it is only a small pinprick, all over and done with in a couple of seconds. But people who are learning how to inject themselves should not be told beforehand that it will not hurt – because that is just not true. Sometimes, it will hurt. Not always, but sometimes.

My reason for saying this is that the person about to do the injection believes that it will **not** hurt. Then, they perform the task and realise that, in fact, it does; but because they were led to believe that it would 'not' hurt, they then feel 'wierd', 'strange', different from everyone else who has had to inject –

... and it 'didn't hurt' ... Rubbish! Of course it did, it's just the people surrounding the person doing the injection are uncomfortable with the concept of pain. Also, the initial, introductory practice of drawing up insulin and practising injections is often performed on an orange. When did you last hear an orange say 'Ouch!'?

The process is unnatural, which is probably why our bodies react by producing a bruise. It is a way of the body showing that it does not like what is being done to it and reminding you, asking you, pleading with you not to do it any more. But what can we do? We need our injections to remain well. If we do not inject, we do not get any insulin, and this can cause an even worse trauma.

The best way round this problem is to devise a rotation system, as we have all heard before, where you only return to any given injection site every x number of injections, and even then it does not have to be in exactly the same spot. This makes sense as it gives the place into which we inject – arm, leg, stomach or wherever – time to recover. We all have to take our injections, we may as well make it as easy as possible for ourselves.

When I started to inject myself in the side and in the stomach, I often noticed annoying little telltale blood spots on my T-shirts. These pinprick stains can also appear on trousers or jeans, especially as we are now told that it is OK to inject straight through our clothes, directly into the thigh. This is another discovery we have to make for ourselves and can cause some people to become even more self-conscious. Who wants to go around wearing blood-stained clothes?

I find it easier to inject my arms and legs. I haven't gone near my backside in ages and I have been using my stomach for injections for quite a few years now. My stomach is the area that becomes most tender after being used as an injection site. I still often wince and hesitate when I inject there. I don't see this as a failing, but I wish I didn't hesitate so much. The injection itself lasts only a second or two, the pain is usually minimal, sometimes even non-existent, but, if anyone touches my side or stomach, I hate it, as that is when it hurts the most.

Sometimes, someone might prod me in the side, playfully and innocently, but my dramatic reaction to this has caused people to give me some funny looks. People do not realise how sore this can be for us, otherwise they would not do it. My arms and legs do not cause the same problems, although my arm sometimes feels 'dead' for a while after I inject it. However, injections have to be done. Mostly, I find it not a great ordeal, but if anything could be done about the soreness that accompanies these jabs we would be most grateful!

4

You 'should' be doing better

I attend my hospital clinic about twice a year. When I was old enough to start going on my own, from about the age of 15, it always struck me that I never saw anyone my own age at the clinic. I only ever saw elderly people, which always made me feel out of place and alone. Often I wondered if I was the only young person in the world with diabetes. Was I some sort of freak because I had it?

Hospital clinic visits were nightmares. You know what it is like: you go in at the appointed time, only to see crowds of people crammed into the waiting room. You report to the desk and give your name and, if you are lucky enough to get a seat, you sit for hours, usually well past the time written on your appointment card.

You become bored and frustrated with waiting. Finally, you are called. You go in, often to be seen by a doctor who hasn't got a clue who you are. Immediately, you are on the defensive. The trusting doctor–patient relationship, essential for honesty and openness, simply cannot exist in such circumstances. As a result you tend to be less than honest with what you say to the doctor. Your only thought is: 'I want to get out of here – now!' So you hold back a lot of the questions you had wanted to ask in your hurry to get it over with. You also find it hard to open up to a stranger, even if they are a doctor. You try to give them the information you think they want to hear, forgetting, of course, to mention your often astronomical blood sugar readings – if you have bothered to do any – or your frequent hypos.

You may get a lecture about your bloods being 'too high' and be told sternly that 'you should be doing better.' It is forgotten, naturally, that life can cause you enough grief without having the worry and hassle of trying to *cope* with diabetes, never mind master it. (Give them diabetes for a week and let's see how they get on!) Just what you want to hear, isn't it? And this is from someone who may know what diabetes is, but who hasn't got a clue what it is to try to live with it.

You might show them your blood-monitoring diary, which you filled in en route to the clinic (forgetting, however, to cover it with convincing spatters of blood). The doctor just cannot understand why your HbA1c result is 15 mmol/l, when you have almost perfect daily blood readings ...

How many of us have gone to hospital for our check-ups and been faced with a young, eager student who tries to be as 'doctor-like' as possible, telling us how much we should eat, how much we should inject, when we should inject, what not to eat ... then cannot understand when we begin to relate the practical difficulties of life with diabetes. They have studied theoretical diabetes for many months, so they obviously know best. What do we know? We've only *lived* with it for years.

How often have you come across the doctor who tells you that you should be getting better HbA1c results? Or how many times have you heard the 'no sweets/plenty of exercise/control, control, control' speech given to you, not as advice, but rather as an accusation? I wonder whether these doctors appreciate how hard it can be to live in the real world and avoid all of its temptations, or even to do everything by the book and yet still not obtain these so-called 'good' results. It's **hard**!

We have to live with the actuality, impracticality and, yes, the threat of diabetes. Don't get me wrong. Student doctors have to learn and many are excellent. If they do not get the opportunity to apply their knowledge, there will be little progress for them as doctors or for us as their patients. But how can they know what it is actually to live and to struggle to cope with diabetes, having only studied the theoretical side for a relatively short time?

Some of the established practitioners, too, really do not know an awful lot about living with diabetes. It is easy to tell someone that insulin must be balanced with a meal, that blood sugar levels should be kept between 4 and 10. I can say that, a child could say that. The problem lies in putting it into effect.

Once I was sent for an eye test. Having never been to this clinic before, I did not know what to expect. Drops were put into my eyes – to dilate the pupils, allowing more light in, making it easier for them to see behind the eyeball. These drops meant I could not see properly for the next few hours, my vision blurred and everything looking extremely bright. My focus was gone and my eyes felt very sensitive. As the drops were administered, I was told what the effects on my eyes would be, and then, almost as an afterthought, the nurse said to me: 'You're not driving, are you?'

Luckily, I was not, but if I had been, how would I have got myself home? I would not have been in a fit state to drive. I felt it was a pity I wasn't warned about it before they put the drops in, just in case I did have to drive.

Then there are the other hospital tests – you know, when you are sitting up in bed in hospital and the consultant brings round a party of students for a tour of the ward, or when you visit your outpatient clinic for a check-up and they call in some other doctor to discuss your case. In these situations you are usually discussed openly, as if you are totally inanimate, as if you are without feelings, worries or even any understanding of what is going on or being discussed. Only it's not you they are discussing, is it? It's the patient, 'the diabetic' they are trying to treat and, what's more, it is the *condition* that is the focus of their deliberations, not the *person* with the condition.

When will it be realised that no two people with diabetes are exactly the same? Though hypos and hypers are encountered by most, if not all, of us with diabetes, my ways of dealing with them may differ from someone else's. If my blood sugar level is raised, for example, I might choose to inject some extra insulin or even inject a larger dose than usual at mealtime, and thus allow myself the luxury of eating something, whereas someone else may just leave things as they are for a while and check later to see whether their level has risen or dropped. If it is dropping, they may decide to leave it alone. If it is rising they may decide to inject more insulin, do some exercise or even skip a meal, if they have the inclination.

'Control' is a word which I am sure everyone with diabetes hears very soon after diagnosis and which is quite an emotive word. Someone who produces an HbA1c result of 6 or under is said to have 'good control'. However, those who get results of over 6 (and I am often in this category) are invariably told that we are 'poorly controlled' or that we do not have good control. We may even be given the favourite phrase and told that we are 'out of control'. Not a nice thing to hear – nor is it very helpful.

We do not want our blood sugars to be raised. Nor do we deliberately break 'the rules', which are often hard to follow and which change as we go along. Life has a habit of interfering with diabetes, just as diabetes can interfere with your life. We do not want to have HbA1cs that affect us detrimentally, but sticking regimentally and rigidly to the impositions which diabetes can bring about in your way of living can cause havoc – psychologically and emotionally, as well as physically. When diagnosed, we're told to take injections, watch what we eat, come back for a check-up in six months 'when we expect everything to be perfect, if not, you are for it . . .'

Diabetes itself can be a cause of loss of control, loss of control of life, especially when it comes out of the blue. If 'control' is so important, it must be given to the person who has diabetes, as well as being in the hands of the medical team. After all, the person with diabetes is the one who has it 24 hours a day, 7 days a week, 52 weeks a year. If the person who has diabetes is not given control of their own condition, then they will not be able to live with it easily.

Both medical staff and people with diabetes must strive to be open and honest with each other, in order for diabetes to be managed well and lived with more successfully. Medical staff must realise that diabetes is an inexact science and will throw up factors that cannot be accounted for as well as strange,

against-the-grain occurrences, even if the theory says
otherwise. Equally, those of us who have the condition must
be open enough to say when we have overindulged, or when we
haven't bothered to do our blood tests, or not taken our
injections, so that we can get the best possible care from our
medical teams.

You will get a lot more out of your clinic visits, provided
of course that they do not condemn you for being honest. If we
do not divulge our secrets, we will not benefit. Don't worry
about upsetting the medical staff – they are supposed to be
there to *help you*, not to put you down for slightly overeating
or feeling too tired or too lazy to take that recommended bout
of exercise.

Diabetes is a very individual condition. While a lot of us
share common traits, such as needing insulin, having hypos
and so on, many things are unique to each of us. Even
though we have the same condition, no two people with
diabetes are exactly alike. For instance, I like sport, am
usually fit and I do not require a great deal of insulin. But
someone else with diabetes may hate sport and, therefore, is
less likely to be as fit and will probably require more insulin
than I do. This does not make me better or worse than the
other person. It just highlights the differences between us –
even though we have the same condition.

This leads me to believe that it is vital for both the people
living with diabetes and the medical teams who treat us to get
to know each other on a more personal level. Why should we be
treated as if we are all the same, when we are obviously not?
What is the use in telling us that we should eat at *x*, *y* or *z*
o'clock, if our life circumstances make it very difficult or
impossible to do so? What is the point in advising someone
to exercise 'at least three times a week' when they have kids
who need to be collected from school, clubs, friends? Or if
there is a relative who needs constant care, or a family
member in hospital?

Treating diabetes is quite different from living with the
condition. In *treating* diabetes, the theory is exact, but *living*
with it – well, anything can happen in life – the theory gives
way to reality.

I accept that doctors, nurses and other health professionals
know a great deal about diabetes, but what do they know about
living with it, day to day? The getting up in the morning and
facing a stomach puncture before breakfast ... and lunch ...
and dinner. The ongoing riddle of how much insulin to add, or
subtract, depending on your routine for that day. Or, in some
cases, the fact that you couldn't care less about the magical
blood sugar figure of 6 mmol/l because of your sister/brother/
parent/job interview/children/bills/funeral you're dreading.

Whenever I am told that my blood sugar 'should be 6'
I want to say: 'You should try to live with diabetes yourself,
just to see what it is like.' I wonder how many medical people
could manage to produce HbA1c's of 6 again and again – or
even once – and at the same time still manage to cope with and
try to derive some enjoyment from life?

We need our doctors and nurses – without them we would
struggle. But we need them to understand just how difficult it
can be to cope with this condition. Each person with diabetes
has his or her own diabetes. What works for me, may not work
for someone else. We may have different lifestyles, certainly we
will have different bodies, and different problem-solving
methods. Maybe that is the message to put across – that
diabetes is as individual to each person who has it as each
person is to any other.

Tips and hints

Depression

People with chronic conditions including diabetes are three
times more likely to suffer depression than the general popu-
lation. Signs of depression include:

- no longer enjoying or being interested in most activities;
- feeling tired and lacking in energy;
- being agitated or lethargic;
- feeling sad or low (downhearted) most of the time;
- weight loss or weight gain;
- sleeping too little or too much;
- difficulty paying attention or making decisions;

- thinking about death or suicide.

According to research, depression in people with Type 1 and Type 2 diabetes may also have the following effects:

- they are less likely to eat the types and amount of foods recommended;
- they are less likely to take all their medication;
- they are less likely to function well, both physically and mentally;
- they are more likely to be absent from work.

Any person with diabetes who believes they are suffering from depression should see their doctor.

5

Eight square meals a day

My first 'real' job was working for a courier company. I started working there in the summer of 1989. The hours were regular, although I began work at 6 a.m. I was office-based and only a half-hour walk or 10-minute cycle ride from home. However, within the first few weeks there, I was having really bad hypos. I was usually smack bang in the middle of one before I realised I was having a hypo. By then, transforming this realisation into positive action, or even communication, was almost impossible.

I must have had some kind of alarm system within me to 'find sugar!' when this happened, as I always seemed to be able to do so. But I went through these very frightening hypos for weeks and I was either too afraid or too embarrassed to say anything to anyone.

I am still not sure what caused this bout of hypos. Perhaps it was emerging from my adolescence? But they may have been caused by my keeping my insulin amounts the same every day, instead of adjusting them. At the time, however, I simply did not know how. Or it could have been due to my method of travel – walking or cycling – and my minimal breakfasts – I am not a great eater first thing in the morning.

They eventually passed, but this may have been due to the increased amount of junk food I began to consume on an almost daily basis – and this was not exactly sensible. At the time, though, with my limited diabetes management knowledge, it seemed to me to be the right answer. Unfortunately, it did not totally prevent hypos.

I worked from 6 a.m. until 1 p.m., then would go home, often back to bed. On occasion, I would have to stay later, so I would have my lunch at 1 p.m. and then resume working at 2 p.m. Usually, I would bring my lunch with me, as I would know in advance when I would be staying on late. But, one time I had no food with me. As it was a courier firm, the drivers were often contacted by radio – in those days before mobile phones – to go to the chip shop and collect orders for lunch, quite a normal and regular occurrence.

Knowing this and not having any food with me, I made my way up to the controller's room and ordered fish and chips for lunch – at about 6 : 10 a.m.! The other staff sat there, stunned and silenced, and then everyone burst out laughing. 'We haven't even had our breakfasts yet, and you're thinking about your lunch!' said one of my colleagues.

This brought it home to me how much in advance I had to prepare – almost half a day, sometimes a whole day – if I was going to be training on a particular night. Another colleague commented that I needed: 'Eight square meals a day.' I don't think he knew just how close to the truth that was.

Once, when I was at work, I felt myself starting to become hypo, so I went into the canteen for a glass of milk. As I was sitting and drinking, someone came in and said: 'Oh, so here you are, skiving off work again.' I realise it was a remark that was not intended to cause offence, but I was trying to prevent a hypo in as dignified a way as possible. I was only in the canteen for a few minutes and I was able to return to work almost immediately, but it struck me that this person's views could be widespread. Are people with diabetes seen as lazy, careless or even manipulative by our friends and work colleagues?

One of my more spectacular and public hypos happened when I was about 20. Just home from work, I realised I needed to get something from the supermarket, a 10-minute walk away, so off I went. I was fine until actually in the supermarket and then plunged immediately into a hypo.

I knew that something was wrong. I may even have known what was wrong. I can even remember picking up a bottle of Lucozade and starting to unscrew the top, until my conscience reproved: 'You can't have that, you haven't paid for it.' I got through the checkout, paying for my bits and pieces, and began to walk home. Even in this state I was planning to cross a dual carriageway.

Luckily, I ran into Liam, a friend of mine, who realised that something was amiss. Perhaps it was my staggering about or the fact that I was being extremely loud and giggly that alerted him. He grabbed hold of me and steered me safely across the road. But the journey home is a complete blank. When I got indoors I was given food and, gradually, I came round.

When Liam had found me, his first thought had been that I was drunk, but then he remembered that I do not touch alcohol. I was so lucky that I ran into him. However, after I had recovered physically, the embarrassment, the guilt, the shame all began to set in – feelings that were almost worse than the hypo itself. I had made a public exhibition of myself. I had shouted goodness knows what at goodness knows whom in my incapacitated state. Luck was on my side in meeting a friend – a short time later I was not so fortunate.

In September 1990 I had just turned 20. I was on two injections a day, mixing medium-acting and quick-acting insulins. I was still uneducated about things like adjusting insulin doses to suit myself, or even about rotating injection sites – all I did was to stick the needle into the left or right cheek of my backside.

One day that September I began to feel unwell. The real sign was my loss of appetite – a sure indication that I was not quite myself. I took a few days off work, doing nothing much – staying in bed or hanging around the house. With my lack of appetite, I was not eating very much. What I was doing, however, was injecting the same amounts of insulin.

The weekend came and I was feeling slightly better and by Saturday evening I decided I was well enough to travel with the swimming club to a gala in Mullingar, County Westmeath. So, on the Sunday morning, I went to the competition. I was actually too old to enter any events, but I had taught a lot of the kids at the club how to swim and I wanted to see how they would get on. Unknown to me, though, a 'teachers' race' had been scheduled and, when I was asked if I was going to enter, I succumbed to temptation, got in and swam – even managing a second place.

When I got out of the pool my appetite, which had almost completely returned before the race, disappeared again, so I ate only a tiny amount of lunch. On the journey home I told one of my friends that I would not be going with him to the Iron Maiden concert, which was planned for later that night, as I was quite tired and had to be up for work at 5 a.m. the next day. I sold my ticket, somewhat regretfully, I have to admit, to my friend's brother.

When I got home, I began to prepare for work the next day. I packed my bag and walked to the shop at the top of the road to buy some crisps and chocolate. It was a minute's walk, if that. Then I began to sink into one of the worst hypos that I have ever had. It is hard to explain, but I can remember many little details about this hypo. I can recall being in a daze walking back from the shop, going up to my room and climbing into bed. I left the light on and my brother, with whom I shared the room, asked why I didn't close the door and switch off the light. By now I was well into the hypo, and aware of it, but I just couldn't express how I was feeling to anyone. When my brother asked me about the door and the light, I can vividly remember feeling really annoyed and just kicking the door shut before getting back into bed.

The next thing I recall was a voice saying: 'He's waking up now' and a very sharp pain in my arm, just between bicep and forearm. A couple of minutes more and I became aware of my surroundings. I was in a hospital, a drip connected to my arm, and my parents were looking at me anxiously as I lay on a trolley in the casualty department of Dublin's Beaumont Hospital.

I don't think I have ever had a fright like this in my life – before or since – and I know that I **never** want to experience anything like it again. It was absolutely horrible – all of my worst nightmares at once, my own private hell. Nothing on earth could ever scare me as much as waking up out of that coma. The last thing I was aware of was kicking the bedroom door shut. The next thing I knew was being woken up in hospital many hours later. I recovered physically within a couple of hours, was discharged and went home.

I was called into the hospital soon after for a check-up, and I discussed what had happened with one of the nurses. She believed that, because I was injecting in the same place every time, the insulin was lodging in one place. It was not spreading throughout my system or working as it should have been. When I swam in the competition I had been very tense, but later on my body began to go into recovery mode. My muscles relaxed, including my *gluteus maximus* (my backside), which was where I had been constantly injecting. So, I then had a week's worth of unused insulin spreading rapidly through my system.

I will never forget that date: 23 September 1990. I won a silver medal, sold my precious Iron Maiden ticket and had my worst ever hypo, all in the space of a few hours. I suppose that I was lucky – blessed even. Can you imagine if the hypo had happened while I was in among a surging crowd of headbangers with a huge sound system drowning out my pleas for help? I do not know what prompted me to sell my ticket, but, ultimately, this action may have saved my life.

I pulled through this episode and I learned from it the importance of rotating my injection sites. I have never injected into my backside since then, though, and I don't know if I ever will again. I learned the value of adjusting insulin doses even though I still had a lot more to learn, and I am very happy to say that I have since heard Iron Maiden play on two occasions, without a hypo in sight!

After this, however, I felt I had to get something sorted out. I didn't want to live the rest of my life in fear of another hypo threatening to ruin everything – diabetes seemed to be doing a fair job in that respect. So it was decided that I should be admitted to hospital for a week. I went into Beaumont Hospital in March 1991 and, during that week's stay, my regime was changed from two injections of long- and short-acting insulins a day to four daily injections – three of Actrapid (see Glossary) before each meal (breakfast, lunch and dinner) and a long-acting insulin, Ultratard (see Glossary), at night before I went to bed. This was the first time I had ever encountered a 'pen' device for injecting. The syringes I had been using were now replaced by a nifty looking pen, designed to look like a luxury writing implement, rather than a crude syringe. I also got my first glucometer, so that I could keep a close eye on my blood sugars and see how much insulin I needed to take. I learned a bit about how to adjust my doses and I felt more comfortable with my situation. I even began to inject the recommended 30 minutes before each meal, although sometimes this was just not possible or practical.

In September 1991 my employers relocated from north Dublin to an industrial estate on the south side of the city. My firm and another merged from two buildings into one, but the new building was hardly prepared to accommodate office equipment, let alone staff moving in.

This lack of preparedness also applied to the canteen and kitchen area. However, the new kitchen did have a microwave, which helped me a great deal. I was in the habit of bringing my pre-prepared lunch with me each day and heating it up in the microwave. This meant I had a regular meal at lunchtime every day. One day, however, I went upstairs, having taken my injection, to find that the renovations were now overwhelming the canteen. Nothing was in its usual place, including the microwave.

Having already taken my Actrapid, I went to heat up my food, only to find that the microwave was missing. I started to look around and ran into the person responsible for the renovations and asked him if he knew where it had been put.

'No.'

I asked him if he knew who had moved it.

'No.'

I told him I needed to heat my lunch, so that I could eat, but his reply will stay with me for ever.

'*You will just have to do without,*' he said.

I was stunned. His attitude was that I – and my work colleagues – could take our breaks without eating. I was too shocked by this response to even argue with him. '*You will just have to do without,*' he said, dismissing me in such a careless manner that it angers me now, thinking about it, more than it did then, having had time to reflect on the possible consequences.

Fortunately, one of my workmates realised what was happening and came over to tell me he had found the microwave and brought it back to the canteen, where I was able to use it and eat. This incident made me much more mindful of the need to make sure I had all the equipment I needed, before I wanted to eat.

Working for a courier firm did have its advantages, though. Once, I arrived at work to discover I had forgotten my kit – glucometer, pen, insulin – the works. I quickly made arrangements to get a courier to call at my home to collect my bag of gear. I rang home to say someone would be calling for my kit and that it was okay to give it to him. Everything was delivered to me within an hour, in plenty of time for my lunchtime injection. When I went home, however, I was told that the courier was an unshaven, leather-clad biker, with rings in his ears, nose and even his eyebrows (well before this fashion was widespread). Even though my family knew someone would call for my bag, they were still highly reluctant to hand it over to this character!

I began to check my blood sugars regularly. I now had a meter to gauge my readings, and, of course, this was very attention-grabbing, wherever I went. At work there was a guy who used to come up to me when I was testing my blood sugars with my new gadget, thrust a fat, sweaty palm under my nose and say: 'Do me.' He wanted me to check his cholesterol levels, as he thought I could do that test for him as well.

One day, in the middle of a heatwave (most countries call it summer – in Ireland, however, sun in July is considered to be a heatwave), my supervisor at work went out and bought 14 choc ices for her staff. It was a kind act of generosity, but when she proffered one to me I wasn't sure whether to refuse politely or eat it. I had to make a decision fast. How bad would it make my supervisor feel if I refused her gift, compared with how bad would it make me physically feel if I went ahead and ate the ice cream. Guess what? I ate it.

I checked my blood, which was around 6 at the time, and it was not too long after lunch, which was a slight help as eating 'treats' after a meal will not make the blood sugar rise as quickly as if the 'treat' is eaten on its own. But later on, when I checked, my blood sugar level had risen to 13.7 mmol/l. It was totally my decision to eat that choc ice, but I felt that there were other external factors that influenced it.

If I had refused, would I have been seen as ungrateful? Would my workmates have seen me as odd, different or even bad? All these thoughts passed through my mind and, finally, I did bow to the pressure, but was it fair for me to feel under pressure from a simple act of kindness? OK, so I am exaggerating the incident into a mini-drama, but even so I **did** feel pressurised and I wonder whether other people with diabetes have similar simple agonies?

I got my first glucose meter, or glucometer, in 1991. Glucometers are designed to check the level of sugar, or glucose, in our blood at any given moment. This has been a great breakthrough in diabetic care and these meters are becoming more snazzy and compact – some are even mistaken for mobile phones. However, when these meters are advertised it is usually by someone with a wide, beaming smile as they happily show off the meter displaying a reading of 6 or 5.6 – the 'perfect' blood sugar reading.

Why don't advertisements for these machines ever show a reading of 17.6 or 2.1 or 'Lo' or 'Hi', which would lend more credibility to their reliability? I mean, if we had glucometers that constantly gave us 'good' readings, well, we'd hardly have diabetes, would we? Also, we might learn to trust the machine a little more.

Many of the meters are good. However, when the same person's blood is tested on two different machines, simultaneously, I have never seen the result duplicated. Even the same machine, performing the test twice within a couple of minutes, using the same person's blood both times, rarely comes up with the same reading both times.

Often the difference is not minimal, but significant. One machine might display a 4.3 while the other might read 7.4.

Fair enough, both readings indicate that there is no great risk of a hypo. But what if a person's blood glucose level is actually **lower** than is being displayed? For instance, if a person's true blood sugar level was 2.7 but the meter gave a false reading of 5.6? This could put the person at risk of a hypo, by suggesting that it is not necessary to eat when, in fact, the opposite might be true. The meters we rely on **must** be accurate – our well-being can often depend on them.

Blood testing brings another problem – sore fingers. After a while, fingers do toughen up, but every now and then I hurt myself in doing a test. As I do a lot of sports training and because I do not always recognise my hypo symptoms, I tend to check myself more than most people. One of the results of this are callused fingertips with black spot marks. Also, I have a habit of going for the same fingers a lot of the time.

I remember being away on one of the children's camps organised by the Diabetes Federation of Ireland (DFI). One of the young girls used the same finger over and over again to test her blood sugars. While I admired her courage, I was shocked at the state of her finger. When I asked her about it, she told me she only ever used two of her fingers. Both had horrible black lumps on them, so I made her promise to avoid using these two fingers for a while!

I always played a lot of football while I was growing up. When I learned how to take my own readings, I always made sure that my blood sugar was well into the teen numbers before I went to play a match. Off I'd go, play, come home – but I could never understand why my blood sugars would still be raised, even after having played football for an hour and a half. It really puzzled me, sometimes even worried me, but more than anything else it **annoyed** me!

Having raised blood glucose levels can actually impair your performance. They can leave you feeling sluggish, tired and lethargic. To the casual observer, it could have looked as if I was not playing well, or that I was not concentrating fully, which may well have been true – I'm sure it was on many occasions. A lot of the time, though, it may not have been down to my lack of interest or dearth of footballing skills – I was actually not a bad player. I may have been playing while hyperglycaemic, resulting in my not performing to the best of my abilities.

I had always been led to believe that exercise brings blood sugar levels down. What usually happened was this: we played in a Sunday league, which meant that 95% of the time we played at 11 a.m., finishing around 1 p.m., then we'd go home. Sometimes, I would do a reading and see a raised blood glucose level, be puzzled and annoyed, have my injection, then around 4 p.m. I would begin to feel a hypo coming on. I did not know then, but this was as a result of my exercising with a raised blood sugar level, combined with taking a 'full' injection afterwards. Later on, when I would take my injection at lunchtime, after playing football, I was combining the insulin with the injection I had taken that morning. As I know now, insulin combined with exercise results in a drop in blood sugar levels, as a person's body can take hours to recover from physical activity. In other words, I was in effect overdosing, leading to my late Sunday afternoon hypos.

This sounds bad, but at times I did not always feel the hypo or its effects. I just knew, from carrying out a test, that my blood sugar was low. At these times I could make the most of it. I could sit down by the fire, watching a football match or a film on TV, relishing an ice cream or a bar of chocolate, without worrying about it pushing my blood sugar levels up too much and most definitely without any feelings of the guilt I usually experienced when I was eating these 'forbidden foods'. A strange type of bliss!

Tips and hints

Diet

Your diet is very important. People with Type 1 diabetes should have a diet that has approximately 35 calories per kilogram of bodyweight per day (or 16 calories per pound of bodyweight per day). Most people with diabetes find that it is helpful to sit down with a dietician or nutritionist for a consultation about what the best diet is for them and how many daily calories they need. It is important for people with diabetes to understand the principles of carbohydrate counting and how to help control blood sugar levels through the proper diet.

Generally, carbohydrates should make up about 50% of the daily calories (the accepted range is 40–60%). Carbohydrates are foods that can be broken down into sugar. They make your blood glucose levels go up. If you know how much carbohydrate you have eaten, you have a good idea what your blood glucose is going to do. The more carbohydrates you eat the higher your blood sugar will go.

Most of the carbohydrates we eat come from three food groups: starch, fruit and milk. Vegetables also contain some carbohydrates. However, food in the meat and fat groups contain very little carbohydrate.

Fat is a nutrient and you need some fat in your diet. But too much fat isn't good for anyone and can be very harmful to people with diabetes. It is very important that you limit the amount of fat in your diet by avoiding fried foods, choosing lean cuts of meat and removing extra fat, by eating more fish and poultry (without skin), by using diet margarine instead of butter, drinking semi-skimmed or skimmed milk and by limiting the number of eggs you eat to three or four a week.

People with diabetes should also use less sugar. Foods high in sugar include many desserts, sugary breakfast cereals, table sugar, honey and syrup. One 12-oz can of a regular soft drink, for example, has nine teaspoons of sugar. It is also important to avoid processed foods as they are often high in sugar and fat, and low in nutrients. And don't waste your money on 'diabetic' foods – they are often high in fat to make up for the lack of sugar.

High blood pressure often goes along with diabetes. High sodium intake has been linked to high blood pressure. So, cut down gradually on salt used in cooking and at the table, and avoid high-salt foods such as crisps, processed meats and tinned soups.

6

You could be worse off!

Once, during a football match, I started to feel as if I was on the verge of going low, so I called over to the sideline to ask someone to get me a bottle of Lucozade. A young lad scooted off to the local shop, bought the bottle and hurried back. I did not want to chase over to the sideline to pick it up. After all, I was playing in defence and my absence might give the opposing team the opportunity to score a goal, so I waited until the ball was at the other end of the pitch, then shouted to the lad to throw the Lucozade over to me. He did, I caught it, opened it up – and was promptly covered in bright orange, sticky liquid.

All the running and shaking had had the obvious effect on the carbonised contents of the bottle, hence my Lucozade shower! There was about half a bottle left, which I drank, enough to let me complete the game. But I wonder what the opposition team thought when I shook hands with them at the end? With my sticky palms perhaps they thought I should have been in goal! My 'going low' during games was an all-too-regular occurrence, and my way of combatting this was the old 'eat more chocolate' method of prevention. While on the whole it helped, it was still frustrating.

Just before my 21st birthday, I began to learn judo, a brilliant sport – strenuous, energetic, and graceful when well executed. I quickly came to enjoy the sport as it required strength, agility, speed, fitness and a positive mental attitude. However, as it was so strenuous, it led me to having quite a few hypos. My way of dealing with this was to keep eating more, often two chocolate bars en route to a tough training session, and more afterwards.

I was still on Actrapid at this time. When I was training, I would have my evening meal of sandwiches around 4 p.m., and then would need to eat chocolate or drink Lucozade about half an hour before getting on to the judo mat. My midday meal was usually eaten around 1 p.m. Because I started to train at 7 : 30 p.m. I preferred to eat my evening meal at least three hours earlier. However, at the time I had to take more insulin to cope with the sandwiches. I should have been eating a snack to cope with the peaktime activity of my midday insulin dose. In effect I was virtually overdosing on insulin when I should have been reducing both the midday *and* evening doses. This was the reason that I was always in need of more glucose just before my bouts of extremely vigorous and tough exercise.

I did have a very encouraging teacher in Paul Cummins. He was very enthusiastic about training. So, I stuck with the sport and enjoyed it, even with the discomfort caused by my diabetes, such as training on a full stomach, and my then lack of knowledge about how to treat the condition.

A judo competition was arranged in Galway, in the west of Ireland. Paul decided to drive us down to Galway from Dublin in a coach. We set off the night before the competition, the plan being to sleep on the coach, when it was parked up, before and after the competition. Cheap? Yes. Uncomfortable? Most definitely. Not only was it difficult to sleep on the bus but, because of my inexperience of judo competitions, I also ate loads of junk food – chocolate, sweets and crisps – the night before the competition. I even chanced reducing my insulin intake that night, because I was so afraid of going low during the bouts. As a result my bloods shot through the roof and, consequently, I needed to go to the toilet every 15 minutes. Except we had no toilet on the coach, which was parked overnight in a car park. After my fourth expedition in the

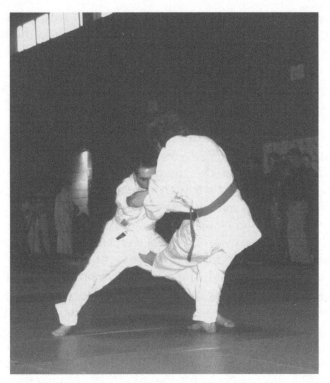

Figure 5   John – Galway, March 1996 (on left, white belt) – he won
this one.

dark, trying to crawl toward the door without disturbing my
fellow competitors, I wondered whether I would have to stand
peeing out of the door all night!

Another time, about two or three weeks later, a gang of us
went on an adventure weekend in Delphi, County Mayo, again
in the west. There were five of us. Delphi is an adventure
centre, where people can take part in such activities as rock
climbing, hillwalking, abseiling and surfing – lots of physical
activity.

The first time that I ever went to Delphi I went with David
and a friend of ours for a week. I decided in my wisdom that if
I was on holiday from work, then I also needed a holiday from
my diabetes – and so I dispensed with my blood testing for the
entire physically-very-active week!! I just went on how I felt

and reverted to the tried and tested method of eating loads – probably far more that I actually needed! I don't know how, but I got away with it – not a hypo felt, nor even any adverse effects from raised blood sugar levels. It was bliss!

The way in which mealtimes operate in Delphi are like this: we would get brought out to do our activity, and when we arrived back we then got our meals. In order to be fed, though, a queuing system operated. So, when you got back you dumped whatever gear you had on in your room and went back down to join the queue – first come first served. Anyway, we were all out surfing one day, but I did not bring my insulin along with me – I did not see any need, as I knew we would be back in plenty of time for our meal. When we got back to the centre the evening meals were already being served and a queue had already formed, so we went up to our room to dump our gear. I also had to get my injection, but the others went back down to join the queue with *We'll see you down there in a minute!*, or words to that effect, shouted over their shoulders as they ran downstairs.

It only took me about 30 seconds, perhaps a minute, to find my injection, take it out, dial up the dose, inject and put it away again before I was ready to go down to eat. So, having done the necessary I went down after them to join them for dinner. However, by the time I got to the queue there was already more people between me and my friends, and I had to stand at the end, apart and away from my group. By the time I had my meal on my tray the others from my group had already found a table, but by the time I was ready to sit down all the other places at their table had already become occupied. I looked for a vacant place, and the only one I could find was at a table at the other end of the room away from my group. I ended up sitting with people whom I did not know and ate my meal within that group while the others from my own group sat together, having a good laugh, discussing the events of the day.

I felt so isolated and in my view needlessly so, as it would not have cost the other lads anything just to hang on for that extra 30 seconds or so, while I injected. I then would have been able to sit down with them and join in the discussions, the joking, the laughter, the fun; but because of their thoughtlessness – albeit unintentional and unconcious – I became separate, apart and felt as if I yet again had been distanced because of my diabetes.

In September 1995 I began a creative writing course. One of our homework assignments was to write 10 words that meant something to us and then to compose a poem containing those words. The word 'diabetes' was on my list of words, and a few nights later I sat down to work on my poem. Within an hour I had written 30 verses.

As I was in full flow, we had a power failure. I hurriedly lit a candle and just kept on writing, such was my desire to get my feelings down on paper. The words just kept on coming, as if a tap had been turned on and allowed to flow. I eventually finished and sat back to read over what I had written.

I had had diabetes for 20 years, but in all that time I had never really spoken to anyone who really understood both me and the condition. I was suddenly expressing feelings that I had kept suppressed for years. It felt so good to get these feelings out. I also began to realise that I needed help to deal with issues that I had raised. I had taken a momentous step – without fully understanding what I was doing.

I found writing a very therapeutic way of helping myself become a more positive person, not just about having diabetes but also about other parts of my life. One reason it was so therapeutic was that no one told me to 'stop complaining' or that I was 'better off than a lot of people' or simply to 'shut up'. No one looked askance as I described blood tests, injections, hypos, comas. It was a totally liberating experience. It also made me appreciate how much diabetes can be an emotional as well as a physical burden.

'Don't complain – you could be worse off' is a shut-up-and-stop-annoying-me comment that usually comes from someone who does not have diabetes. Sure, we could be worse off – but we are entitled to have the opportunity to air our grievances, disappointments, worries and fears. It is easy for someone without diabetes to say that we could be worse off – but how would these people cope with the condition, I wonder?

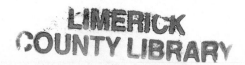

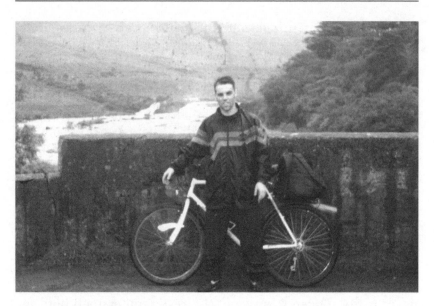

Figure 6   John – Delphi, Co. Mayo, circa 1994.

I was diagnosed with diabetes aged just four years old on 15 May 1975. Over the years, I had known feelings of anguish, pain, guilt, fear and shame. I often felt alone and isolated. Not until 20 years later did I realise that I had never – **never** – spoken to anyone about how I felt having diabetes, living with it, struggling with it and, quite probably, dying with it. I suddenly felt the urge to find someone who would not only listen to me but who would also really **understand** me. I needed to know that, when I expressed myself, I was being understood.

But where could I go? To whom could I turn? The answer came through an advertisement in *Balance*, the magazine of the former British Diabetic Association (BDA), now known as Diabetes UK. This particular advertisement was for a weekend away with people aged between 18 and 30 with diabetes. I rang and asked if I was eligible to attend, as I came from Ireland. Thankfully, I was accepted and I made arrangements to travel over to England. This was one of the best decisions of my life – the weekend I went on was a truly life-changing, life-enhancing experience!

7

Famine to a feast

It was a bit scary, leaving Ireland and arriving at Manchester Airport all on my own, but once I had touched down there was no turning back. I boarded the train for Stoke-on-Trent and began to feel the butterflies all over again.

I arrived at the hotel venue in Stoke and checked in at the British Diabetic Association's (BDA) Youth Diabetic (YD) stand. Panic was about to overwhelm me when a guy strolled up and introduced himself. He seemed about my own age, friendly and relaxed and I began to relax too. 'What's this weekend all about?' I asked him. 'Have you been on one before? How long have you had diabetes?' Questions I was to ask over and over again throughout the weekend. Questions which I was also asked, in turn. By the time the introductory meeting for first timers at the YD weekend was due to begin I was feeling a lot more confident.

After the meeting – an informal and relaxed welcome to all the newcomers – we went off for a tea break. Feeling braver, I began to chat with some of the others. The ice was now well and truly broken. I knew I had taken a big step, and it was beginning to feel as if it was paying off.

At dinner that evening I will never forget the overwhelming feeling of **belonging**. For the first time in my life I was **not** the only person in the room having to take an

injection before I ate. Virtually everyone I looked at was
doing the same thing. I will never forget that moment.
I knew I was not on my own in the world, which I had often
felt until then. I felt good, relieved, relaxed – I did not have to
launch into my usual explanation about what I was doing and
why I was doing it. In fact, it looked and felt so **natural** to be
injecting, a feeling I had never experienced before. Previously
I had always felt different, now I was just the same as
everyone else.

The YD weekend was structured around discussion groups
and information workshops for young people with diabetes.
The discussion groups encouraged people to talk about
anything that was troubling them regarding diabetes. The
information workshops were run by health care professionals
with a good knowledge of diabetes or by young people with
diabetes.

There were groups on travel, sports, relationships,
complications, insurance – everything I had always wanted to
know but had either been afraid of asking or had been
prevented from asking in the past. It was incredible – for the
last 20 years none of these questions had been answered for me.
Now I had come from a famine to a feast!

Often, during the discussions, I would think: 'Hey, that
could be me saying that.' Or: 'Wow, I thought I was the only
person going through that.' A huge burden was lifted from me,
just on hearing that there were others who had experienced the
same troubles, difficulties, fears and emotions which I had
previously imagined only I experienced. I kept telling
myself: you are not alone. You are **not** alone!

As the weekend came to a close, we went our separate ways.
I swapped addresses and phone numbers so that I could stay in
touch with my new friends. What's more, I also got in touch
with Simon, the guy who had come up to me at the start of the
weekend and helped me settle in.

Simon wrote back, telling me he had been happy to help,
and he invited me to keep in contact. We are still in touch, but
when we meet now we rarely discuss diabetes! We have a lot of
other things in common. Julie, his wife, told me that it was
quite uncharacteristic of him to go up to a complete stranger

and start to talk to them, without an introduction. I have a belief that we were destined to meet.

Now, whenever I go to any meetings like that one, I always recall my first time and the fear and panic, and I try to talk to those who are there for their first time. It is daunting, it is a challenge, it can be quite scary – but, believe me, it is worth it.

I went back to Manchester Airport to catch my flight home, and, because I had a 5-hour wait for the flight, I decided to ring home. I dialled the number.

'Hello, where are you?'

'I'm at Manchester Airport, on my way home.'

At this point I was overcome with an intense desire to cry. Only as I said I was on my way home did I realise how far away I would be from my new-found friends. At the YD weekend I felt as if I **belonged** somewhere. Now I had to leave and I did not want to go. I had not wanted the weekend to be over. I wanted it to go on and on and on. I felt so good just by being there.

I think there were a number of factors that provoked this reaction. In Ireland, at that time, there was nothing like this available. There was no one my own age to whom I could relate as easily as I could to those at the YD weekend in England. I felt a real part of this group, and it was a wonderful feeling which I did not want to end. For the first time in my life I had been happy because of my diabetes, instead of being hurt by it.

THEY DIDN'T DESERVE IT – LET THEM IN
May, Nineteen Seventy-Five
Fifty-Six months alive
Life soaring, took a dive
When we found out

Always thirsty, always dry
Unlike the other boys
Even though he tried and tried
Not to want so much

To the doctor I was brought
A curing remedy was sought
But of my breath a whiff he caught
And to hospital he sent me

'Diabetes' we were told
And it turned my parents cold
Heavenwards their eyes rolled
I too young to understand

'You must stay here for some days'
Somebody was heard to say
With whom now could I play?
As I stayed six weeks

In my arms and legs they stuck
Nurses held me as I shook
My life gone (as I mistook)
I did not like it there

For six weeks I stayed put
Little boy, mouth shut
I would love to go, but
I had to stay there

Insulin was pumped in me
Legs as sore as sore could be
But no one my pain did see
As I wept myself to sleep

At last I was free, out
Happy Day! Joyous Shout!
Left, however, in no doubt
That this was for ever

Time and time I returned
To the place my stomach churned
A time that I wished burned
Out of my memory!

Some time later, very thin
Face gaunt, pale skin
Hospital – I went back in
To be re-taught the rules

Six years later, struck again
This time not too much pain
Fortunate, or I'd be insane!
I thought I was in 'control'

I surfaced some time later
Wondering how I could cater
Still no girlfriend – I no dater
No one to really share this with

Then one day I read
Magazine advertisement:
'*YD Weekend, Stoke-on-Trent*'
Opportunity to be availed of

Day of journey, my heart beating
No need – friendly greeting
Now came my time for meeting
Others who could really comprehend my anguish

Problems shared, problems lessened
Sharing made them less unpleasant
Easier now, others listened
Whom I *knew* could understand

Maybe we were made this way
To make it easier on Judgement Day
For GOD to Look at us and Say:
'THEY DIDN'T DESERVE IT – *LET THEM IN!*'

By then we will have the right
To feast with GOD in all His Might
Without the worry, or the sight
Of injections digging into us to allow us to eat

(John Keeler, 17 April 1996)

8

Steering my own ship

I came home from England a changed person. I saw just how good the Youth Diabetic (YD) weekend had been for me, and I wanted more. But how could I get more? There was nothing like it available in Ireland – would I be forced to move to Britain? I even considered this for a while, but then thought: why should I have to move so that I can access something that should be available to me at home?

I began to go to more meetings arranged by the former Irish Diabetic Association (IDA), now called the Diabetes Federation of Ireland (DFI). I also started to attend information sessions which were organised by local branches of the IDA. One meeting was a launch of a local branch. I went, listened and, toward the end of the meeting, I asked about the possibility of setting up a youth section. I told them briefly about my trip to England and wondered whether it would be possible to set up something similar in Ireland. 'That's a great idea,' they enthused. 'Good luck in setting it up!'

I was utterly frustrated by this response. I believed the IDA should be providing this sort of service, yet the organisation was clearly hoping that I would organise it for them! I went home very disillusioned. The YD event had completely changed my life in a most positive way. I had the same feelings and problems as those young people I had meet in Stoke-on-Trent, but they had the benefit of regular meetings, friendly shoulders to cry on, easy access to each other.

What about those of us in Ireland? What had we got? I continued to go to IDA meetings. I wasn't especially interested in somewhat depressing talks on how blind I might become in a few years time or how my feet were in danger of falling off because of gangrene brought on by diabetes. Both of these are risks, true, but I do not expect these problems to happen to me. Why should I? I am fit, healthy and generally look after myself. I went to the meetings, though, in the hope of coming across other young people with diabetes and then maybe something would happen.

One night I drove out to a meeting in Tallaght, in the south of Dublin. At this meeting I first met Gráinne, who was about my age. We made beelines for each other, and after briefly talking about ourselves and our experiences with diabetes we swapped phone numbers and began to keep in touch. I told her about the YD weekend in England and she decided that she would go over to the next one, a few months later.

I had been in touch with one of the small group facilitators from the previous YD weekend and she had written back, encouraging me to facilitate a group at the next meeting. I put my name forward, was accepted, and was invited to attend a training weekend. The training was directed by two psychologists and I found it fascinating. It also made me realise that not everyone with diabetes has the same view of the condition.

To facilitate means to make easier – and that was my intention. I wanted to make things easier, not just for the small group with which I was working, but for anyone I came across, especially the newcomers. It doesn't cost anything to be nice and a friendly welcome goes a long way to helping someone to relax. Once they relax, everything else becomes so much easier.

Gráinne came over to that weekend too, her first experience of YD. We had an agreement that, as we knew each other, we would not spend the whole time together. The idea was to get to know as many new people as possible, and this helped us both in making new friends while we were there.

When I came home, I again went to as many meetings as I could. At one, the IDA was looking for young people aged between 16 and 26, with diabetes, to take part in a challenge – to climb the highest mountain in each of Ireland's four provinces within 36 hours. The intention was to get the message across that people with diabetes could do whatever they wanted.

This challenge was to take place in August 1997, and in order to get fit I began to run a lot in the evenings. I am not a great fan of running or jogging – I find it boring and it does not do my knees any favours. But it is a cheap and relatively easy way to build up fitness. Cheap in that I only needed a pair of trainers, shorts and a T-shirt, and easy in the sense that I did not require expert tuition in order to run.

I liked to run in the field at the bottom of my road, just five minutes from home if I ever felt a hypo coming on. Having a goal to aim for kept me focused and made me push myself a bit harder when running. Often I would come home from work, and even though I really wanted to lounge in front of the TV I would keep the Four Peaks Challenge in mind and make myself get out there and run.

I was still on Actrapid at this time and began to experiment with reducing my insulin doses. I would cut the insulin dose before my evening meal, sometimes by up to 50%, wait the recommended half-hour before eating and make sure my dinner was not too heavy a meal. Then I would wait for a couple of hours before doing my stretching exercises, check my blood sugar levels and go for my run.

One evening as I was about to start stretching, I did a blood test, which read 4.3 mmol/l. I thought about sitting down and watching TV or reading a book for the evening. But there was nothing on TV or a book I was eager to finish, so I decided that I really needed to go for a run. I felt fine, so checked my blood sugar again, about half an hour after my first reading. This time my reading was 5.4 – my levels were beginning to rise. I thought that if my bloods were on the way up, it might be a good time to run – so I did.

I ran and did some other exercises, spending around 45 minutes out in the field. When I got home, I checked again – 7.3. This was above the level at which I had begun my bout of exercise, but a perfectly acceptable level by anyone's standards. What had happened was, as the Actrapid 'peaked', the blood sugar began to rise. This coincided with my beginning to exercise. So, even though I was exercising with a rising blood sugar level, there was still sufficient insulin present to cope with the exercise and the rising blood sugar.

This was a really useful discovery to have made. It meant that, by manipulating my injection doses, I could eat less before I exercised. It also meant I did not have to eat chocolate before exercising, if I did not want to. I continued this method of eating/training from then on, and it has really helped both my performance and my diabetes. I still make mistakes now and again, but on the whole I am able to adjust my doses of insulin. I also became more confident about **not** eating at times when I felt that food would interfere with my participation in sports. Progress was being made!

During summer 1997 the IDA arranged for those of us participating in the Four Peaks Challenge to meet regularly to get to know one another and to practise our climbing skills. We climbed each mountain – a great way to spend a summer while getting acquainted. There were nine of us with diabetes – Orla Wilson, Orla McCarrick, Andy Brown, Nigel Kielty, Dave Augusta, Dave Barrett, Kieran Flanagan, Fergal Cronin and me. It was brilliant to be able to do an activity as strenuous and enjoyable as mountain climbing, in the knowledge that everyone around was aware of our diabetes. We did not have to keep explaining about the condition.

We also had a medical team: doctors Chris Thompson, Adrian Daly and Randall Hayes and nurses Helen Twamley and Caitríona Coleman – Caitríona also happened to have diabetes. A lot of learning took place, not only by those of us with the condition. The medics also learned quite a bit.

By the time Saturday 30 August came round, we were all fit and raring to go. Accompanying us was a camera crew – a television documentary was being made about our efforts.

The plan was to tackle Ulster's highest peak – Slieve Donard, 852 metres – where the Mountains of Mourne do indeed sweep down to the sea. Then we were to be whisked away by helicopter to Mweelrea Mountain, 819 metres, on the rugged Atlantic coast of County Mayo. We would then fly south to Kerry, where, the following day we would take on Ireland's highest mountain and one of its toughest, Carrauntoohill, 1,040 metres, before finally flying up to Lughnaquilla, 926 metres, in County Wicklow.

According to our schedule, we were to commence climbing at 6 a.m. on Saturday and, by 6 p.m. the following day, we would be standing on top of Lughnaquilla, having climbed a total of 3,637 metres and made a round trip of some 438 miles. Our challenge was to be made into a television programme, to be shown nationally. We felt we had a responsibility to do ourselves justice.

I had to concentrate, not only on my performance but also on my physical condition at every given moment. I felt I had to make sure this was going to turn out successfully. I cannot recall any other time in my life when I became so focused, so single-minded and so prepared, physically and mentally. I was running five days out of seven and, on three of those days, I was also doing circuit training, as well as running. I even resisted playing football in case I sustained an injury which might prevent me from taking part in this great event.

I also swam, which was excellent for keeping fit and also for staying injury-free. I had also grown much more comfortable in adjusting my insulin doses. A team of diabetes-specialist medical advisers had given us new ideas during our training climbs. I had found ways of reducing my Actrapid by sometimes as much as 60%, of not eating chocolate and of timing my training so that I did it just as my bloods were beginning to creep up. Mistakes were becoming fewer and further between.

We had to get up at 4:45 a.m. on the first day of the challenge. I was shivering when I woke. Cold? Or excitement? I dressed quickly and went down for breakfast. Double helpings all round and don't ever believe the myth of a person not being able to eat three Shredded Wheat! Some of us had four or five. We stuffed ourselves in preparation for the difficult task ahead.

We checked our blood sugar levels and, for once in my life, I was disappointed to see 6.1 registering on my machine. I had cut my insulin intake at breakfast by 50% and had eaten a larger than usual meal. I really could not comprehend this 'perfect' score. We gathered for a photograph and then, after being counted down, we were off, climbing Slieve Donard before the sun had risen. There was no going back now.

As we climbed, I ate Jelly Babies until my bloods began to rise. We stopped at various points for a breather and to carry out blood tests. About a third of the way up, we had a break for food, gazing down at the sun-kissed sea below. It was simply breathtaking. With just one more stop, we reached the summit at 7 : 55 a.m., well ahead of schedule. We stayed there a short time, to eat and take some snapshots. On the way down, the camera crew flew over in a helicopter, reminding us of how we were to travel on to Mayo, a trip we all eagerly anticipated.

I also noticed something else. I was **bursting** to go to the toilet, which puzzled me. Had my bloods risen so much after I had just climbed a mountain? When I checked my blood sugar level, it had risen to over 23! After my significant insulin reduction at breakfast, I had then had a big meal, in anticipation of the intense amount of exercise. In addition, I had continuously eaten chocolate and Jelly Babies while climbing. Obviously I had overdone it.

The insulin/exercise alliance was being defeated by the large amount of glucose and carbohydrates which I had consumed, leaving me needing more insulin. Even at this stage I was still making errors, but also learning that in order to do anything in comfort, my system needed some insulin. Climbing the mountain had not really taken too much out of any of us, so I looked at my options for the rest of the climbs: reducing the insulin intake by a lot but not eating too much junk food, or reducing the insulin intake by a smaller amount – up to 35–40% – and tucking in to the chocolate, sweets and biscuits.

I happen to enjoy a lot of junk foods; so, I chose to reduce the insulin intake by the smaller amount and enjoy feasting on treats. After all, it wasn't too often I could feel comfortable eating chocolate and sweets in front of our diabetes-specialist doctors and nurses. I just could not let the opportunity slip by!

When we got down the mountain, we restocked our bags, had something to eat and then boarded the choppers for our first flight in a helicopter. We got to Silver Strand in County Mayo and began the ascent of our second mountain of the day at around 1 : 20 p.m. Mweelrea was very wet and boggy, and it took a lot of effort to climb. However, by 4 : 30 p.m., we had conquered it and, as yet, not a hypo in sight.

Then it was on to County Kerry where, next day, we would take on Ireland's biggest and best mountain Carrauntoohill. That evening I really enjoyed my meal – and for a special reason. By the time we started to eat it was 8 p.m. I had had three Actrapid injections already that day and I was unsure as to whether I should inject more to compensate for my new intake of food. I had managed to get my blood sugar level back under reasonable control by then. It was around 10. I asked one of the doctors what he thought, and he said that I should be OK to eat without injecting again. I didn't need to be told twice! That night I ate my first meal in ages without having to inject insulin beforehand, and under medical advice too. I was absolutely thrilled. I really enjoyed not having to inject – it meant so much to me and I'm sure those of you on insulin will know what I mean.

We went to bed at 11 p.m. – and, yes, I did take my night-time injection – and then were woken again at 4 : 30 a.m. to prepare for the next leg of the task. When I checked my blood it was still only 10.3, the combination of extensive exercise and my night-time insulin (at this time I was on Ultratard) had kept my blood sugar level from rising excessively.

Rain was pelting down as we left. It was so clouded over that we had to wait until 6 : 45 a.m. to set off, over three-quarters of an hour later than planned. We were already behind schedule and, on a day like this, time was going to be precious. Climbing the part of the mountain known as the Devil's Ladder was tricky enough in good conditions. It was a much more muted group that set off this second morning. We walked for the best part of an hour before we reached the foot of the Devil's Ladder, the real start of the ascent of Carrauntoohill. Everyone was already soaked from head to toe by then.

As for blood tests ... well, you will have heard of random blood testing. On this day we invented *tandem blood testing*! Fergal and I stopped to check our bloods, but, as it was raining so hard, we had to take it in turns to shelter each other while we tested. Any rainwater on the blue testing strips would dilute the blood and would give inaccurately lower readings. We were so wet when we were doing the tests that we had to assume that whatever result was displayed was lower than our actual blood sugar levels. So, when my meter told me my blood sugar level was 7.6, I guessed it was actually around 12 or above.

Ascending the Devil's Ladder was tricky, too difficult for our camera crew who could not manage to carry their equipment as well as negotiate the tough, steep climb. We kept going, but were now climbing up through a virtual waterfall, created overnight by the unremitting rain. We were like salmon! Blood testing was out of the question – we just went by how we were feeling and kept on chewing.

At 9 : 45 a.m. we reached the top of Carrauntoohill, smiled briefly for photographs and then began to descend. I was beginning to feel extremely cold and started to become concerned about my well-being. The climbing had kept me warm, but once we stopped I began to freeze. I managed to keep myself moving until it was time to go down, and as we began our descent I munched away at my sandwiches. As we had to be extremely cautious coming down, we fell even more behind schedule. Also, because of the low, thick cloud we were informed that the helicopter flight to Wicklow would be slower than the previous day's trip.

Soup and more sandwiches were waiting for us on our return and we needed to change our sodden clothing – still more delays. As we boarded the bus at 12 : 30 p.m. we felt unsure about whether we would meet the 6 p.m. deadline. Then, one of our guides, Sean Sweeney, turned to us and delivered a truly inspirational speech in his broad Kerry brogue. Sean said that, if he had possessed just half our 'tremendous spirit, courage and determination', he would have stood on top of Mount Everest long ago.

The mood on the bus instantly changed to one of hope and optimism. I don't know if Sean realises what he did for us that day, but he told us exactly what we needed to hear at exactly the right time. Thank you, Sean. We now believed we could climb the final mountain. But did we have enough time to do it?

One of our group suddenly had a really bad hypo. It was bound to come. There had been a few minor worries over the past two days, but nothing that a gulp of Lucozade or a mouthful of sweets or chocolate could not solve. Now, one of our colleagues could not remember coming down the mountain he had just climbed. Some of the group helped him through it, feeding him, staying with him and talking to him, and it was not long before he was back 'with us'.

None of us now doubted that we would reach the top of Lughnaquilla, but how fast would we progress? Worrying would not get us to Wicklow any faster though, but praying might ... which is what I did. By 3:20 p.m. we had touched down and began the final ascent of our fourth mountain in just over 33 hours. By this time I was becoming quite emotional. I felt a lump in my throat, but forced myself to concentrate on the final push, promising myself I could be as emotional as I wanted when I reached the top.

The group was beginning to spread out now. Our race against the clock had become a battle. We stopped briefly for blood tests – my blood was around 7, so I had the last of my Jelly Babies. As we got closer to the summit, enveloped in clouds, our only thoughts were whether we would make it before 6 p.m. I was in the first group of six people and the rest, although not far behind, were still behind. We had started as a team, we had to finish as one.

The Wicklow Mountain Rescue Team members who accompanied us from the bottom of Lughnaquilla were a Godsend, so were their walkie-talkies. We were able to ascertain how far behind our colleagues were. Suddenly, they came into view, once more raising our hopes and spirits. It was now 5:30 p.m. One more rock face and then a few steps to

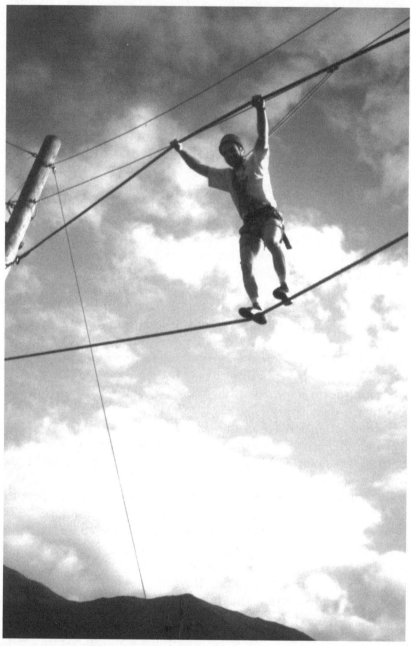

Figure 7   The difficulties of maintaining balance
(John – Delphi, Co. Mayo, circa 1999).

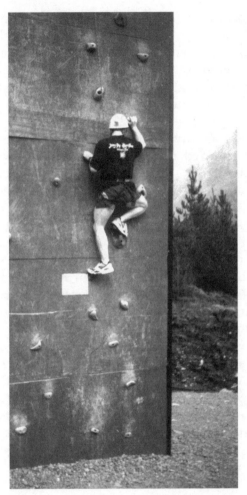

Figure 8   Life with diabetes: full of ups and downs
(John – Delphi, Co. Mayo, circa 1999).

create – for me at least – a new way of thinking about diabetes.
Even our camera crew had managed to make it in these
atrocious conditions, to capture our final moments. No one
gave a thought to blood sugars, whether they were up, down
or flying around, we were too busy getting ready to finish what
and how we had started – together.

   We lined up next to each other and joined hands.
At 5:53 p.m. on 31 August 1997 we conquered the fourth

peak of our Four Peaks Challenge – finishing with 7 minutes to spare. The conditions were awful, but we overcame them all to show that life with diabetes, though often a struggle, can still be a fantastic adventure.

As we jumped around for joy, I gave thanks to God who had sustained me, not just over the previous two days but through my 27 years – over 22 of them with diabetes. I buried my face in my hands and cried. For more than 22 years I had endured this condition. I lived with it as it harassed and hindered me, restrained and shackled me, tortured and abused me. It had delivered some cruel blows – physically, emotionally and psychologically. It had kicked me when I was falling and held me down as I tried to rise. But now I **knew** I could do anything that I wished to do. Diabetes no longer had to rule my life. Sure, it would always warrant consideration, but many other things in life need the same. I was so happy and relieved by the successful conclusion of our great adventure. My body had proved to be in good shape – it was now up to my mind and spirit to catch up.

Being involved in the Four Peaks Challenge was another huge and positive turning point in my life. It made me realise that, although I could not push diabetes aside, I could fit it in to what I was going to do. I did not have to let it dictate my plans. It is part of me – and always will be – but its position has changed from navigator to passenger. A new, better stage of my life began at the end of the Four Peaks Challenge. I had at last come to terms with living with diabetes. I was steering my own ship.

(A BIT MORE THAN) SPANCIL HILL
Last night as I lay dreaming
Of (dubiously!) pleasant days gone by
Me mind, bein' bent on rambling
Through Four Peaks I did fly
We stopped on board a chopper
And forced against our will
To climb four Irish mountains:
Donard, Mweelrea, Lughnaquilla and Carauntoohil!

It being on the 30th and 31st of August
The same day as the U2 concerts
Where Ireland's sons and daughters
And friends assembled in Lansdowne Road
But we, nine young diabetics from Ireland
Had a duty to fulfil
Climb four mountains in 36 hours
Including Carauntoohil!

I went to see me neighbours
To try to raise some money
Some looked exhausted at the thought
Some just signed and paid
The I met some generous people
Who sponsored from their till
And I'm sure we'll need someone to mend our breeches
When we finish these four 'Hills'!

We paid a flying visit
To Mweelrea from Slieve Donard
Neither as white as any lily
Nor gentle as any dove
We cast our eyes upwards, saying:
'We've two more mountains still
Lughnaquilla is last tomorrow (Thank God!)
But next is Carauntoohil!'

I dreamt I fell and blistered
Which obviously was quite sore
'Ah Johnny, are you low? – Have some food
Or Lucozade – here, have some more!'
Then the meters showed improvement
From *'Low'* to *'10'* and rising still
We awoke dreams in diabetics by climbing
Donard, Mweelrea, Lughnaquilla and Carauntoohil!

(John Keeler, September 1996)

9

That!!

With my extra knowledge and new-found confidence, I went from being someone who had been reluctant to discuss diabetes to being almost an in-your-face person with diabetes! I began to see my situation and that of other people with diabetes in a different light. For example, have you ever met people who believe you should inject your insulin out of their sight? You know, the people who say: 'You should go to the toilet to do that.'

For years, I would disappear into the lavatories to save having to explain what I was doing and why I was doing it. When I think of some of the revolting places I have visited in order to carry out my injections, it makes me shudder. We are constantly exhorted to wash our hands and to keep the insulin vial and injection sites clean and free from infection. As people with diabetes, we are thought to be more prone to infections. Why, then, have we retired to the toilets for years to inject? Fear? Embarrassment?

There was a time when we did not all have pen devices. We had to use a vial and a not-very-attractive syringe. I don't know how many times I have been in some horrible, awful toilets, pretending to be 'normal'. A way of trying to enhance the portrayal of this normality was to flush the loo, emerge from the cubicle (after having injected), then proceed to wash my hands (if there was a sink and soap available!).

Think about it. You go and wash your hands after completing the injection. Surely doing the injection in a cleaner environment than a toilet area would go a long, long way to eliminating the risk of infections in the first place!

Sometimes, you will meet people who, on seeing you inject or test your blood, will exclaim: 'I could never do **that**!' The emphasis is always very firmly on the word **that** and manages to express real disgust. Those of us with diabetes never considered having to do **that** either, until it was forced on us. **That** is something we now have to face on a daily basis. But **that** is not a pleasure for us either. Some day, they too may have to do **that**, not just once but over and over again. So, instead of saying: 'I could never do **that**', why don't they try thinking: 'What if I had to do **that**?' and see how they feel?

Once, in a cafe after training, before I ate my sandwich, I produced my pen device and took off the top, displaying the needle. A woman at a nearby table hissed at me: 'Surely you're not going to do **that** in here?' I just calmly injected myself, replaced my pen in my bag and asked if she had a problem with it. She replied that it was 'disgusting' and should not be done in front of anyone else. Well, I was off. 'Because **you** are uncomfortable with it, you think **I** should disappear then?' I asked. 'How do you think I feel about it? It's not as if I enjoy doing it. I have to do it, to stay healthy.' I did not really want to have an argument, but I felt that if I did not stand up for myself I might as well go back to scurrying down to the unhealthy, unhygienic lavatories for ever more.

I now inject publicly and unashamedly. I have often in the past had to deal with being called a 'junkie'. No matter how many times I hear it, it never ceases to annoy me. I don't smoke. I don't drink alcohol. I take lots of exercise. In other words, I try to look after myself as much as I possibly can. Diabetes was forced on me – I did not have a choice. In order for me to stay alive, I have to take injections. Using the word 'junkie' implies that we do the injections for fun, for kicks, to get a 'high'. How wrong could they be?

Then there are the blood tests. 'Ugh. Take it away,' is a

frequent response. Well, it's not exactly a bundle of laughs for us either. We do not enjoy being human pincushions. And then there are the people with diabetes in TV programmes. The 'diabetic' is either comatose from having astronomical blood sugars or has collapsed due to a really bad hypo. In the end they are usually saved by the hero doctor. Why can't a person with diabetes be shown in a more positive light?

I have nothing against people with diabetes being portrayed as sufferers – there is some truth in it – but having diabetes does not mean constant suffering. So, how about creating a character who has diabetes but who can be admired? What about showing a diabetic person who has the normal ups and downs of life, but who still gets on with it?

Often, a diabetic character will be shown injecting into a vein in the arm. We inject into our upper arms, our thighs, our backsides, our stomachs. But, we inject **subcutaneously** – under our skin – **not** intravenously – into our veins. It does not take very much research to find this out. If a person with diabetes is going to be portrayed, they should be portrayed more realistically. There is a lot more to diabetes than knock-you-out hypos and hypers.

Perhaps some of the terminology used should also be changed. For instance, when our blood sugar readings are below 4 mmol/l of blood, we have been taught to refer to them as being 'low'. When they are above 10, they are 'high'. Two friends with diabetes and myself were on a train, chatting away, when we decided to check our blood sugar levels. The readings on each of our machines ranged from 13 to 17 and one of us remarked casually: 'Oh, I'm high.'

We all produced our pens for some extra units of quick-acting insulin, when I suddenly became aware that we were doing this in full view of the entire carriage-load of people on the train. I knew by the look on the face of an elderly woman that she thought we were drug addicts. So, I began to chat about diabetes in a loud voice, to allay any fears that we were abusing drugs.

If we were taught to use the words 'up' or 'raised' instead of 'high', this would improve matters, I feel. 'High' is associated with being high on drugs. 'Up' or 'raised' is not and are more positive words that would take a lot of the stigma away from people with diabetes. It is a small change to make but one that could create a positive change in attitudes toward us.

There is so much lack of awareness out there. I recall a time when I went to someone's house on the way to go training. As I waited for him to get ready, his mother asked me various questions about diabetes – I think I had just done a blood test.

'*How often do you have to inject yourself?*'

'I'm on four injections a day now.'

'*Oh – you must have it **really bad** …*'

A classic!

It did, however, highlight to me the misconceptions and lack of understanding and knowledge of our condition.

10

Living on my own

After we had successfully accomplished the Four Peaks Challenge and after my trips to England, I was a much more confident person, especially where my diabetes was concerned. I was also much more open with people about it, because I had come to understand the condition much better. I was more willing to talk to people about it and spoke of it in a more informed way. When it came up in conversation, I spoke with much more authority than before. I felt, for the first time in my life, that I almost had complete control of it. However, there was still one thing that was missing.

I had always hated going to hospital. It brought back so many painful memories. Most of all, I hated feeling as if I was wasting my time at the outpatient clinic. I would sit in an overcrowded room for hours until I was finally called into the doctor's room, either to endure another lecture about how *bad* my control was or else for them to go through the usual routine of *name/age/dosage* while never once taking their noses out of the chart, just as if it was a quiz, but one in which if I failed I was condemned to yet another lecture ...

'*Name?!*'

Of course I know my own name, you idiot!! What a stupid question!!!

'Age?!'

I think I'm going to *scream* ...

If they were really interested in knowing my name and age, surely they would look *at me* when asking, instead of at that horrible chart as if it was a cross-examination, as if they were trying to catch me out! It also might help if they *asked* me instead of using accusatory barks. And as for those record books ...

Record books are the books in which we 'record' our blood sugar levels after we have done our tests. Or: *do we?*

I remember a doctor at the Youth Diabetic (YD) weekend talking to a group of assembled diabetics about how well aware he was of who had recorded the *actual* blood sugar reading, as opposed to those who had just filled them in *en route* to the clinic.

How did he know?

Easy ... by the amount or, rather, *lack* of blood stains on the pages! And, I have to admit, he was correct. I – and I am sure many of us – have pulled that stunt on occasion or even regularly.

Picture the scene: someone who does not record their blood sugar levels in their monitoring diary, either because they could not be bothered or do not feel the need to, or even because they do not do any tests anyway, on their way to their appointmtnt with the consultant (*and an entourage of students*) at the clinic. They realise that there is nothing in their diary to show the doctor, and think: *'OH, SHIT!! I have nothing to show in my record book!! – I'd beter fill it in!!'*; so, the diary is then filled in, usually with 'excellent' results. If they have any guile, every now and then a raised blood sugar level will be recorded, and maybe the odd low here and there, just for the sake of balance. It will then be produced for the doctor's perusal, who may look at it approvingly but who will then be at a loss to explain the HbA1c of 14 which has come back ...

It is like copying the homework that you did not do the night before, and hurriedly getting something down on paper just prior to the teacher wanting to look at it!

Why is this done?

Well, for my part, when I used to do this it was to avoid being lectured about keeping my blood sugars down at the ultimate, golden level of '6'. I did not like being angrily told that I *'should be doing better'* (it sounds more like a teacher–child relationship the more I go on), especially by someone who did not have to even contemplate trying to keep their own blood sugar levels from rising too much.

It felt like going to a trial where I was both victim and criminal all rolled into one, where even though **I** was the one suffering, **I** was made to feel that it was all brought about by my own doing, that it was all my own fault.

What utter, nonsensical **CRAP**!!

It also felt as if I was reporting to a parole officer or going to someone who had the power to make me feel better by no more than a nice remark or a smile, yet knowing in my heart of hearts that all I was going to get was a '**GUILTY!**' condemnation from a finger-pointing judge and jury in the guise of a doctor who had not got a clue who I was and who in all probability would never see me again.

I have gone through phases where I have religiously recorded every blood test along with any exercise I have taken and how much insulin I have injected. I have also had my fair share of times when I have just tested and injected without recording my life in that little white diary. I can see one good point about recording my personal (diabetic) information, and it is mainly related to any time when I enter a new routine in my life.

For example, when I changed over from Actrapid insulin to Humalog insulin (in late 1997) I recorded absolutely everything. I even tested an hour after eating once or twice, just to see how well the Humalog acted. I have found it personally beneficial to record my insulin amounts, times of injections and blood sugar readings before and after, say, any time I go training. From recording my insulin intakes and readings I could judge where and when I got it right and where I went wrong – al I had to do was look back at my diary and take it from there. I could see where I took too much insulin or where I ate too much, or where I did not inject enough insulin. Because I recorded everything, my

diary became a reference book for *me*, and me alone. All I had
to do was to look back at what I had done in any similar
situation, compare my readings of the time with those of the
previous situation and proceed according to what had
happened the last time: if I had gone hypo I would take less
insulin that last time, or eat more, or combine both solutions; if
my blood became raised after the exercise I would take slightly
more insulin than last time, or eat less, or possibly both.
Recording can be a hassle, but it became a very useful tool
for me – and most times it was a good guide.

It came in very useful both before and during the Four
Peaks Challenge, during which I got to know Dr Chris
Thompson and he got to know me – who I was and what
sort of lifestyle I had. So, soon after our climbing adventure,
I changed clinics and became his patient.

In order for people with diabetes to receive proper and
informed care, a good, honest, open relationship must be
established between those of us with diabetes and the
medical teams we entrust with a share of the management of
our condition. I now feel I can have a much more open and
honest discussion with all members of the medical team. I am
also now much more willing to listen to them.

I got to know the team mainly from attending weekends
away organised by the Diabetes Clinic at Dublin's Beaumont
Hospital. These weekends brought together people of a similar
age who all had one thing in common – diabetes. These
weekends were different from the YD weekends in England.
The Diabetes Clinic weekends focused on learning about our
diabetes through participation in physical activities, whereas at
YD weekends there was more talking, but little actual exercise.

At the National Adventure Centre in Tiglin, County
Wicklow, a group of younger people with diabetes took part
in such activities as hill walking, rock climbing, abseiling,
gorge walking and kayaking. It was refreshing to look around
during a hill walk, for example, to see that most of the other
participants were doing blood tests or taking injections – just as
I had to do. Even after my experiences during the Four Peaks
Challenge, I still got a kick from seeing other people doing
what I was doing!

Frank, meaningful exchanges took place over these weekends and we had structured group discussions as well. My facilitator training was utilised to help, inform and support people who were encouraged to know that they were no longer alone. Experiences were shared and everyone learned something. Both those of us with diabetes and our medical team became much more informed about what it is to **live** with diabetes. Friendships were formed, myths were dispelled. Everyone came away with a better and more thorough understanding of their diabetes and more honest interactions between 'diabetic person' and 'medic' were created, with the result that we got better care and a better grip on our conditions. Many thanks are due to the Beaumont Clinic for all they have done for us. I am grateful and I know the other participants are too.

These weekends helped to heighten our self-reliance. One of the big concerns of people with diabetes is becoming so incapacitated by a hypo that we may have to rely on others for help. This concern is exacerbated if we are away somewhere where no one knows we have diabetes, or if we live alone. If a large-scale hypo occurs, what do we do?

If I go to bed when I am low and do not necessarily feel it, my body's reaction is to refuse to allow me to sleep. If I do manage to drift off before becoming low, I will wake up without any of the drowsiness that usually accompanies waking from sleep. I will go from being asleep to being wideawake within a couple of seconds. I may not always feel as if I am hypo, but I have learned to recognise this type of sleeplessness as a warning sign that I am in fact low. I keep a bottle of juice or a sugary drink in my room, in case I cannot get to the fridge.

This sudden waking seems to be a common sign that a hypo is approaching, or has arrived. I know I am not the only person to have experienced this sensation, but I do not know if it is a universal trait among people with diabetes. However, it could be worth bearing in mind that, if you are finding it hard to get off to sleep, it **may** be because you need to eat.

When I first moved away from my parents' home, I moved in with people who had no experience whatsoever of any aspect of diabetes. I found myself explaining to my new housemates about me and my ways, telling them not to be worried if they saw me jabbing needles into myself, and about hypos and what to do in the event of my having one.

Even so, I knew I needed to be totally self-reliant, as my housemates would not always be around; a lot of the time I would be home alone. Staying on top of my diabetes became even more important. During my initial settling-in period, I kept my bloods raised slightly, and knowing that I would be alone in the house at times made me really conscious of controlling my blood sugars. I knew that if anything did happen to me there would probably be no one for me to call on for help. I began to keep bottles of Lucozade in my room and to eat toast or bread before going to bed. I even began to wear my medical identification necklace when I was alone in the house, in case anything ever did happen.

I remember being invited to a wedding of a schoolfriend, who was getting hitched in the Netherlands. I was looking forward to the occasion but slightly scared of going to a country where I did not speak a word of the language. This was the first time in a long while that I had been worried about my diabetes. What if I had a hypo? Would I be able to communicate that I needed help? After all, hypos can cause slurred speech, aggression and fear, all of which could be a problem if I was seeking help. If I went too low, would anyone know what to do?

I arrived in Amsterdam and boarded the train – but missed my stop. This meant I was going to miss the evening meal – that was all I needed! I eventually arrived just as the plates were being cleared away. I was welcomed very warmly, and as I was about to launch into my 'I have diabetes and I need to eat' speech the sister of the bride-to-be said, in perfect English: 'Oh, I have diabetes too.'

You have no idea how relaxed I became. This meant that I did not have to go through the endless explanations and could just get on with what I had to do. I knew there was someone else there who had to go through what I did. It was a huge help – and I had a great time at the wedding too!

I began to get to know a colleague from work and told him

of my diabetes and how I was living away from my family. He changed jobs and moved from Dublin, but we kept in touch. Later, when a number of people with whom we had both worked gained promotions a big night out was planned. My friend said he would like to come up for the evening and I agreed to let him stay with me.

My friend had often heard about my injections, but he had never seen me execute one. As I went to do my night-time jab, I first checked my blood sugars so that I could decide how much insulin to take. My reading was about 11 mmol/l and I took 18 units of Humulin (see Glossary) insulin, knowing that this would be enough. As he watched, my friend asked about my glucometer, the readings, the amount of insulin – the usual questions. I explained that if I did not eat then – we were having tea and toast – after having injected myself with insulin, my blood sugar level would be very low in the morning, which would not be good.

He then asked a question I have never forgotten. 'Are you sure you will be OK?' I was not sure whether to laugh or scream with frustration! This was someone who knew me and who was aware of my myriad physical activities, such as swimming, hill walking and judo, and who openly admired my fitness. He **knew** that I could look after myself – yet here he was asking me whether I would be OK. In other words, he was saying: 'Do you know what you are doing?'

This guy had asked for my advice on training and diet – now he was questioning my ability to look after myself. In the end I had to laugh, and when I explained why I was amused he had the grace to look a bit sheepish. At least I knew I had someone to look out for me!

11

But this is the hand
I shoot with ...

All my life I have been an active participant in sport – football, swimming, judo, hill walking, circuit training, running and lifesaving. As a child, however, it was mainly football and swimming. In 1975, when I was diagnosed with diabetes, I was put on one injection each morning, which had to cater for all my diabetic needs right through until the following morning.

There was nothing I liked better when I got home from school than to go out and play football, after I had done my homework. Often, though, I'd have to leave early on in the game as I regularly went low and felt weak and extremely hungry. I would do my utmost to stuff myself full of food as quickly as I could so that I could get back to the game. If I ate enough beforehand, however, I would be OK and would not have to leave mid-play to get something to eat.

So, all through my childhood, my adolescence and into my twenties, I got into the habit of eating loads of food so that I could continue my activities without stopping. Often, however, I would eat ridiculous amounts. One night I ate three bars of chocolate to get me though a training session. On Sunday mornings, too, I would do the same so that I could play my Sunday League match without having to be taken off.

It was only at a much later stage that I began to check my blood sugar levels – I was 20 before I got my first glucometer – but even then I could never get my head round the fact that I would often get readings of 14 or 15 mmol/l or above **after** the match. It used to drive me mad! Then, one day, I happened to read an article which explained that if people with diabetes exercise with a raised blood sugar, where there is a lack of insulin then blood sugars will actually rise. This was astounding news to me. I had never heard that before and a lot of things began to fall into place.

Over the years I have usually been swimming before breakfast three mornings a week. When I first went along I was nervous about getting into the pool without having eaten anything. I got into the habit of closely monitoring my readings, which I did just before and immediately after training. I discovered that my blood went from 9.7 before I got in to 13.5 afterwards, even when I had not eaten. One morning I decided to inject one unit of Humalog (see Glossary) before going to train. I ate nothing, swam and discovered my bloods had dropped – but only by a margin of 1 or 2. Interesting.

I was then told that drinking carbohydrates during our training sessions would help maintain energy levels and would also serve to rehydrate the body, without giving me an upset stomach. So, I brought in my powdered carbohydrates, mixed with water in a plastic bottle, and drank it during sessions. When I checked my bloods again after getting out, I found that the difference between the initial reading and the post-exercise reading was often only slight – just a millimole or two.

I was further getting to know my own body. Once, when I had no powdered carbohydrates for my drink, I brought a bottle of water along and swam as usual, with my unit of Humalog inside me. Afterwards my bloods had only dropped by about two points. I have not looked back since making these discoveries.

I have made mistakes, of course I have, but I have a back-up plan of simply getting out of the pool and having something to eat to hand. My love of swimming and my desire to be fit win the day.

I also noticed that whenever I ate Chinese food my blood sugars would rocket. I tried increasing my insulin intake. Most times I injected 10 units instead of my usual 8, an increase of 25%. This, however, seemed to have no effect – my bloods would still head skyward after a Chinese meal. One day I decided to inject 16 units – double my usual dose. It worked! I made sure I was near back-up food when I did this, but I didn't need anything. My bloods did not rise too much at all.

If my bloods were already raised before I ate a Chinese meal I would inject 20 units, with the usual precautions, and this was also successful. This experimentation led me to try increasing my doses *slightly* if my bloods were up before any other meals. Again, I found I was having continued success. As a result, I became so confident about increasing or decreasing my own doses before different sorts of meals or in different situations that I ceased to have a 'fixed' dose. I inject what I need based on activities – done and to be done – and food – eaten and to be eaten – and blood sugar levels.

I **love** to swim. It is a brilliant sport, which does not have to be competitive but which requires technical ability and maintains fitness. I have been swimming since the age of eight years, and in my teens I taught children how to swim and also qualified as a lifeguard. When I began to learn judo, swimming took a back seat for a while. However, eventually I became less active in judo and began to swim again three or four times a week.

The pool where I swam was on my way to work and training started at 7:15 a.m. until 8 a.m. Afterwards I would either go straight to work and have my breakfast there or go to a local cafe with some of the other swimmers and have breakfast with them. I found that my diabetes was easier to manage if I did my exercise in the mornings – though I know this is not always an option for a lot of people.

When I get up in the morning to go training, I check my blood sugar level. I will inject a unit of Humalog if it is over 9 and not bother if it is below that. It might mean an extra

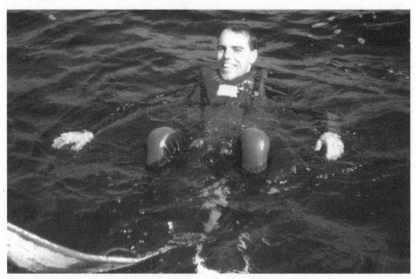

Figure 9   Don't let diabetes pull you under
(John – Delphi, Co. Mayo, circa 1999).

injection a day but not necessarily extra insulin. I might inject a
unit before training, but at breakfast I will only take 4 or 5
units, instead of having one big injection of 8 units, as I do
in the mornings when I am not training. Because I have a
routine, it helps me to regulate my bloods and insulin intake,
as does my fitness level. Also, because I train in the morning
my 'recovery' takes place over the next few hours. If I had an
evening training session, it is likely that soon after I would be
asleep and would be unable to keep an eye on my blood sugars.

When I began morning training, it was a great learning
experience for me to monitor my blood over the few hours
following the training session. I found that if I took my usual
amounts of insulin after training my blood glucose level always
dropped soon after my breakfast. So I knew that to prevent this
I should cut my insulin intake. I also knew that my night-time
insulin was quite effective. So, if I did play soccer or go for a
run or a swim in the evening, it was also wise to cut my night-
time insulin dose, to prevent middle-of-the-night hypos.

My blood sugar levels on the day following training tend
to be lower than when I am not training regularly. This tells

me that exercise is a key element in achieving and maintaining lower blood sugar levels. It also improves fitness
which, in turn, makes lower blood sugars easier to achieve
and maintain.

Knowing how much or how little insulin to take can be
tricky. Unfortunately, there is no set formula – diabetes is
such an individual condition. What works for you may not
work for me, and vice-versa. What activity I have been
doing, or am about to do, combined with my blood sugar at
that particular time, usually makes me decide on my insulin
intake.

When I go swimming, for example, I won't inject any
insulin if my level is below 9, nor will I eat. After swimming
I'll check again. By then it is breakfast and time for an injection
of insulin. If I have trained hard for an hour before I sit down
to eat, I know that the insulin will combine with the training, so
it is like having **two** lots of insulin – from the injection and
from the effects of the recovery period. If I inject eight units of
Humalog after training and before breakfast, it is the
equivalent of injecting 150% of quick-acting insulin. A hypo
will then be looming on the horizon.

I swim for an hour, check my bloods afterwards and inject
only four or five units of Humalog after the swim and before
breakfast – this, I find, is the best way for me to control my
blood sugars. Most of the time, I get an acceptably low reading
later on. If I get up to go training and my blood is above 9, I will
inject a unit of Humalog, not eat or drink any carbohydrates,
then swim and then do what I have described from breakfast
onward.

Why do I inject one unit before training? Surely that would
lead to a hypo? Well, no, actually. If your blood sugar level is
raised and there is no insulin present, the blood sugar level will
rise even further when you exercise. In order for your muscles
to get energy (sugar) from your blood, a certain amount of
insulin is needed to transport the sugar from the blood into
the muscles. If it is not present, the sugar stays in the blood – as
the 'door' through which it must pass has not been opened by
the 'key' of insulin. It is just like when you were first
diagnosed: you were producing no insulin, resulting in

abnormally raised blood sugar levels, meaning you had diabetes.

If my blood is between 4 and 5, I will almost always still swim but only if I feel up to it, or if I have eaten or drunk something with carbohydrates – orange or apple juice, or even milk. It does not bother me too much to swim at these lower levels as I know that most times, due to the lack of insulin and the carbohydrate intake, my levels will rise – or at least not drop too low for comfort. I also know my own body and its reaction and that I have a fairly good level of fitness, which I can trust to see me through.

If, though, my blood is below 4, I will rarely train. I will just go and have my breakfast with probably less insulin than I would have on a normal non-training day. All of this works most of the time for me. It may work for you too, or it may not. I found out through trial, error and recording.

When I changed over from Actrapid insulin to Humalog insulin in late 1997, I recorded absolutely everything. I even tested an hour after eating once or twice, just to see how well the Humalog was performing. Personally, I have found it most beneficial to record my insulin amounts, times of injections and blood sugar readings before and after any time I go training, for example.

From recording my insulin intakes and readings, I have been able to judge where and when I got things right – and where I went wrong. All I had to do was to look back in my diary and take it from there. I could see where I had taken too much insulin, or where I had eaten too much, or where I had not injected enough insulin. Because I recorded everything, my diary became a reference book for me. All I had to do was look back at what I had done in a previous, similar situation, compare my readings from that time to the current situation and proceed according to what had happened last time round. If I had had a hypo last time, for instance, I would take less insulin than then, or would eat more, or combine both solutions. Recording can be a hassle, but it has become a very useful tool for me – and most times it provides a very good guide.

I am aware that not everyone enjoys exercise or is

particularly adept at sports, but if you look hard enough you will find an activity that suits you. The trick is to find something you enjoy doing – and I don't care how much of a cliché that sounds, because it is true! Exercise then becomes something you can look forward to, rather than something that must be done. Go on, you may discover something which you love and at which you also become good.

In the course of my swimming training I have discovered the best levels to have my blood sugars, so that I can train hard and train well. In an average session of 45 minutes, I prefer to have my blood somewhere between 8 and 12, and the session would normally consist of a swim of 1,500–2,000 metres, including recovery swims – slow swimming to get one's breath back. At swimming galas, the longest distance I would swim is 100 metres – the 100 metres individual medley (four lengths of a 25-metre pool comprising one length butterfly, one length backstroke, one length breaststroke and one length front crawl). A fellow competitor once described this as the 'headbangers' event'. Having done it a few times I now know why! This takes me about 1 minute 26 seconds.

There is no real reason to have soaring blood sugar levels if the most I am going to do in any one event is 100 metres. Sure, it takes effort and tires me out, but rarely to the extent that I need sugar directly after the event. I expend much more energy in training than I do in competitions, as I tend to go in for the shorter, sprint events, which do not take as much out of me as does a training session. I see no reason to have bloods that are through the roof. I find that anything around 7 is enough for me at galas. I always have sugar available, of course – as you know, anything can happen!

On 1 January 2000 I fulfilled a burning ambition. I had made a New Year's resolution to swim 50 metres butterfly, a stroke which I love to watch, especially when executed expertly, but which I had still not mastered over this distance. To swim 25 metres of butterfly did not present a problem – it is the first leg of the individual medley. So, I knew I could swim one length. Two lengths, however, were a challenge.

The first thing I did when I got to the pool on 1 January was to dive in and attempt it – without any warm up. I just dived in and swam. Toward the final few metres of the second length – I train in a 25-m pool – I struggled and splashed a bit, but I got there, much to my own personal satisfaction and delight. Later that month I competed in a 50 metres butterfly event at a gala for people over 25 years. So, by the end of January, I had fulfilled another ambition – to compete in a 50 metres butterfly race. I was really pleased with myself, even if my times left a lot to be desired and loads of room for improvement.

Each summer in Dublin there is a river event that has become a real tradition – the Liffey Swim. This is a race from the Guinness Brewery by Heuston Railway Station down to the Custom House, a distance of about a mile and a half. In order to qualify to swim in this race, a swimmer must complete a number of races in the sea swim calendar. In training, I was swimming the required distance at every session and I felt I would be able to have a go at the Liffey Swim.

I went out to swim in the sea a few times, just to get used to being in the sea rather than a pool. It was obviously much colder and much rougher with waves and currents. But I began to go out regularly, every Sunday, for several weeks before the sea swim season kicked off and I was able to spend longer in the water each time I went.

On the day of the first race in the sea swim calendar in June, I went with my friend Liam to the Bull Wall on Dublin's northside, paid the race fee, stripped off and stood waiting for the start. Liam also expected to swim but was not allowed to take part as there was a problem with his registration. So, I asked him to walk alongside me, as I swam parallel to the Bull Wall, carrying my plastic bottle of carbohydrate drink, which he was to throw in to me if I needed it. However, I felt confident that I would not be needing it.

I had purposefully overdone my carbohydrate intake that morning, as well as sufficiently reducing my insulin intake. I had been overcautious in my preparations for this race.

I had never spent so long in the sea, nor had I ever swum a mile race continuously before. Training was always broken into sets of 100 or 150 metres, so I was used to being able to stop. That was not going to be the case on this day.

The water was absolutely freezing, but I soon got into a steady rhythm. Once I was moving, even though conscious of the cold, I felt strong enough to continue swimming. When I swim, I naturally turn my head to the right to breathe. This enabled me to see Liam, walking along the Bull Wall, my bottle in hand. I also saw my parents, who had come down to see how I was getting on. I then noticed, as I swam, that I was pushing fairly big, lumpy things aside with the armpull of my stroke. I wondered what they were – then realisation dawned. They were jellyfish – hundreds of them – and here I was swimming right through the middle of them.

For a split second I panicked, but then admonished myself: 'You are OK. You haven't been stung so far. Keep going, you're OK.' And it was true. I was not being stung and my stroke, while slow, was still in a steady rhythm. I was conscious and aware of everything: the coldness of the water, the huge presence of jellyfish, the amount of time I had spent in the sea – and that, if I really wanted to get out, I was only about 15 feet from the rocky sea wall . . . .

And that was exactly what I did. I got out. I stopped swimming, shouted up that I had had enough and that I was going to get out and swim the short distance to the edge of the rocks that formed the wall. Through all of this I had remained pretty clear-headed, lucid and calm – but things began to change as I clambered out.

'Are you OK?' asked my dad, who had made his way down to the water's edge to help me out. He thrust a branch at me, which I grabbed. As I climbed out my legs began to buckle beneath me. Even now, I still don't know how I got out. I vaguely recall someone draping a fleece over my bare shoulders as I began to stumble toward the car, where I had left my clothes.

'Are you OK?' I heard this question again and again, but I just could not answer. My hearing was fine, but try as I might I could not respond. Liam handed me the bottle of carbohydrate drink and tried to help me put the top into my mouth, but I still could not relax my jaw enough to open it.

'Are you OK?' This question kept on coming and I kept trying to answer, but simply could not. I was still very, very cold, and as I stumbled painfully over the rocks in my bare feet the question 'Are you OK?' came yet again. Suddenly, I was able to scream: 'I'm freezing' (I also swore at him), as we reached the car. [A real sign of a hypoglycaemic person is totally uncharacteristic behaviour – as this was for me! I don't swear, but in this case I did – but it showed the trouble I was in. Also, it may help to explain unreasonable, uncharacteristic behaviour in people which can be brought about by severe hypos.] I had had the sense to pack a flask of hot tea and someone poured me a cup. My arms were shaking like jelly and I had no strength in them at all. Perhaps you have seen the film *Blazing Saddles* and can remember the scene where a guy is describing how steady his hand is. As he is saying the words he brings his hand across the screen and you can see it is trembling violently as he says: 'This is the hand I shoot with.' If you remember that you will know what sort of condition I was in.

As I warmed up I took more food and drink and eventually got my bloods back up. I had also brought emergency food with me, and within a few minutes I had demolished it. In the car on the way home I quizzed Liam about the events leading up to my massive hypo. He said he had noticed a sudden change in my pace and thought I had then become so slow he was contemplating drinking the contents of my bottle and then throwing it to me to use as a buoyancy aid!

I could not understand why I had become so hypo so suddenly, given that I had overloaded on carbohydrates and vastly reduced my insulin intake before the swim. A week or so later I went to hospital for my check-up and I related the incident to Chris (Thompson), telling him that I could not understand why I had gone so low so quickly. I asked him if I had been hypoglycaemic or hypothermic. He then told me about the effects that cold, especially shivering, can have.

Shivering uses up a lot of energy. When it occurs, the muscles are rapidly and constantly contracting and moving, so the actual effort of swimming, combined with shivering as soon as I got out of the water, both played a part in causing this spectacular hypo.

I was lucky – I got out of the water before the hypo began. Even though it was a nasty, horrible experience, I have learned from it. I was previously unaware how much of an influence cold can have on a person with diabetes. Now I know. I still swim in the sea, but I only stay in the water for 10 to 15 minutes at a time, which for me is plenty. I also never swim alone. It was a tough lesson to learn, but learn it I did.

Tips and hints

Exercise

Regular exercise can improve insulin sensitivity in Type 1 diabetes. It plays an important role in reducing other health risks and in managing weight. But care is needed so that physical activity doesn't lead to worsened control.

It is essential to consult the health professional helping you to manage your diabetes before starting an exercise pro-gramme, especially for treatment adjustment advice.

On the day of exercising, evening and bedtime doses of insulin may need to be reduced, as the effects of exercise on glucose control can last up to 12 hours. Take a blood glucose reading before starting exercise. The reading should then stay within 5 and 15 mmol/l. It is advisable to have a small amount of food or glucose drink roughly every 20 minutes, to stay within these levels. Check your blood glucose level immediately after exercise and regularly afterwards. Extra carbohydrate may be needed at subsequent meals and snacks to top up blood glucose.

The five-times Olympic rowing champion, Sir Steve Redgrave, has shown that diabetes should not be a barrier to exercise. Many other people with diabetes take part in the London Marathon every year.

If you have diabetes, however, it is always best to be aware of your limitations and to take precautions:

- perform different activities to exercise different muscles and allow recovery time;
- always begin slowly and build up to a comfortable pace;
- tell someone where and how long you are going to be;
- check your feet after activity, always change your socks and wear appropriate footwear;
- rest or take it very easy if you feel unwell;
- insulin injection sites should be away from the area used during activity;
- remember that delayed hypos can occur up to 36 hours after exercising.

12

Egg-sized potatoes and a cupful of crisps

When I wrote my poem about my life with diabetes, I released a lot of emotions and feelings which had been suppressed for years. Until I attended my first Youth Diabetic (YD) weekend, I had received no help in dealing with these feelings. Perhaps if I could have dealt with some of them sooner, my life would have been altered, possibly for the better. I had carried strong and, often, quite negative emotions about diabetes since childhood. Maybe if I had been able to deal with these my life would have been different. I believe I could have benefited from having someone who would really listen to and understand me.

I was a very young child when I was diagnosed with diabetes, and back in 1975 this meant I spent a great deal of time in hospital, away from my parents and brothers, which left a huge impression on me. I believe these early experiences sapped my confidence and made me less assertive and less able to try new experiences. However, this may have been beneficial in some aspects – I was always too scared to try cigarettes and alcohol!

I have also had a different kind of relationship with my brothers, all younger than me. They knew there was 'something wrong' with John and that he had to be 'looked after'. I was never the typical 'older brother' to whom younger siblings might look up. I accepted the role of the submissive younger brother and even began to accept any misfortune as 'mine'. I thought that was how life was. **I** had to stick needles into my legs. **I** had to stop playing football to eat in the middle of matches. **I** had to endure the name-calling at school.

I **felt** different, and this resulted in my believing that I **was** different. When I was at school, for instance, I was friendly with many children but *had* very few real friends. Maybe I was trying to please too many others in a search for acceptance. As a teenager, especially at the swimming club, I was the one who was at the fringe of it all, who got on well enough with everyone but who did not have a real friend. I went through my teens and into my 20s without forming a real one-to-one relationship with a girl.

Since I came back from my first YD weekend in Stoke-on-Trent, I began to get more involved with both British and Irish organisations. I was regularly in touch with the Irish Diabetic Association (IDA), now the Diabetes Federation of Ireland (DFI), and was told of a planned adventure weekend – the Four Points Challenge, like the Four Peaks Challenge but not as tough.

This was to be a weekend of physical and mental challenges for young people with diabetes from both sides of the internal Irish border. In August 1998 a group of 12 young people aged from 18 to 28, all with diabetes, travelled to Garrison, County Fermanagh, where we met a similar group from Northern Ireland. The weekend involved teams competing against each other in physical and mental tasks. The winning team would be the one with most points at the end.

This weekend was to provide the nucleus of a youth/young adult movement for people with diabetes in Ireland. However, only a small group of people seemed to be interested. To my mind many more people had to be reached.

It remains a mystery to me why more fresh, inter-ested or even curious new faces were not coming along to such events. We went to Garrison for three consecutive years, each year offering a different challenge and genuine learning through enjoyment and self-discovery.

I had facilitated groups at YD weekends in England. On one weekend a participant said to me: 'You're good to talk to', making me feel useful and helpful. I decided to learn counselling skills. I felt relatively confident about the advice I was giving but wondered if it was being imparted in the right way. I also wanted to become more confident in my ability to listen.

I am not suggesting that every person with diabetes should be counselled. However, it is nice to have the option of talking to someone who has been in the same position and also not having to go into all the technical explanations of what hypos are or what insulin does. From doing the counselling course I learned a lot about myself and I felt much more confident about my own abilities to listen and understand. I did not just do it for myself, though, I did it to offer support to anyone who wanted or needed it.

At the first annual children's camp run by the DFI, I was delighted to go along as a helper. In July 1999 we went to Lough Dan in County Wicklow to spend five days with 18 children, all under 14 years, all with diabetes. This was the start of something that is continuing to grow. I think it is extremely useful and helpful to the children who have attended these camps – and their parents.

At the first camp you could see changes in the kids who had come along. I felt happy to be – in a small way – responsible for helping these positive changes to occur. The kids actually talked about having diabetes. What's more they talked to each other about it. Their own experiences were discussed and shared. Why was this so important?

For a start they knew they were not the only ones in the world with this condition – that removed the isolation. They also shared their hypo stories, their blood test recordings, their insulin types and amounts. They moaned about or praised their hospitals, doctors and nurses in an environment where they were not criticised, nor dissuaded from doing so. They had debates about the merits of one type of glucometer over another. They saw everyone else around them doing blood tests, injections, having various types of hypos and having huge readings that went off the scale. The difference was that all this had become taken for granted. This was **normal**.

It was normal for these things to be going on. They could have whole conversations using 'Diabeticspeak'.

'I'm 7.3. You?'

'2.8. That's why I'm going to eat a bar of chocolate. What's your excuse?'

'Very funny. What did you take at dinner?'

'12 Mixtard.'

'Right. Maybe you could decrease it by two units tomorrow.'

'Two?'

'OK then, three.'

And on it would go, making perfect sense to those in the know but gobbledegook to an outsider.

On the first night of the first camp, the leaders kept an eye on things. One of our duties was to test the kids' bloods, regardless of whether or not they were asleep. If we discovered a child whose blood reading had dropped, we woke them and gave them something to eat. This meant that I and the others were in a position to prevent a child from having a hypo.

One time we went to test a sleeping child. The light had been turned off, and not wanting to wake the kids we worked by keeping the door slightly ajar and trying to make do with the light from the corridor. The child we were about to test then rolled over in bed, just as I was about to prick his finger! We had to manoeuvre ourselves around to the other side of the bunk and then work in almost complete darkness. We finally managed to extract the required drop of blood and spilled it into the meter to determine whether feeding would be necessary. Believe it or not the boy did not wake up. I asked the following day whether he had remembered our testing him in the night and he said that he had not felt a thing.

Kids can be amazing characters, especially when given the freedom to express themselves. Often, though, they are not always given the credit which their intelligence deserves. During the first camp, a group of the older kids were in their room, chatting away. The leaders were in the kitchen, clearing up, when one of the group came out to tell us that a girl in the room had become very quiet and was not responding to the banter. A nurse went in and had a look at her, then tested her blood. She had become hypo and the other girls in the group had both the presence of mind to notice it and to react quickly to get something done.

Exchange lists are quite common in dietician's rooms and in diabetes clinics. The lists give a carbohydrate value for different foods. For example, a potato is worth 10 grams/two exchanges, a slice of bread would be the same. If you wanted to eat a certain amount of carbohydrate, but you did not want to eat a potato, you could consult the list to find out what it was equivalent to – such as a slice of bread – and could substitute that instead.

During the first week in Lough Dan our dietician came in for some criticism from me. She had posted one of these exchange lists on the wall for the benefit of the kids. Fair enough, but some of the descriptions of food amounts were ridiculous, I felt. A slice of bread was, for instance, equal to an 'egg-sized' potato. Egg-sized potato? A slice of bread was also the equivalent to a 'cupful' of crisps. A **cupful** of crisps? How many of us eat crisps by the cupful? Why not say a packet of crisps? It makes more sense and is less open to interpretation.

I attended my fourth British Diabetic Association (BDA) YD weekend in Liverpool in April 1999. I had been asked to do the introductory meeting for the newcomers – those for whom YD was a first time experience. I was really pleased to have been asked because I remembered only too well how nerve-racking my first time had been. However, I was nervous about standing up in front of the group and addressing them.

An hour before the meeting was scheduled to start a couple of pages of notes were thrust under my nose. 'Here are your lines.' 'My **what**?' One of the facilitators had written a sketch between two people with diabetes, one 'devilish', the other 'angelic'. Dave Banks (a friend and fellow facilitator) and I were to perform this sketch – at an hour's notice. I had been nervous enough up to then, I was reduced to jelly now! We went up to our room for a rehearsal, then off to the

introductory meeting where we performed admirably ... OK, adequately ... All right, we were woeful! Well, I was. Dave was quite in his element. It did at least get them smiling, which was the main thing, even if it was at our expense!

In January 2000 the DFI launched its video *Juvenile Diabetes: An Information Guide*, an award-winning video, made for parents, teachers, guardians and coaches of young people with diabetes. It features many youngsters with diabetes and has interviews with kids, parents, teachers and coaches about the impact diabetes has had and how they cope with any problems they face. One of the kids featured was a young girl whose mother was interviewed at the side of a swimming pool, while her daughter swam.

Seeing another common link besides the diabetes, I decided to get in touch with the family. I was invited out to dinner one evening and off I went to meet the Ross household, taking along some of my swimming and judo medals. My aim was to encourage young Lindsey to keep going, keep trying and not to let diabetes get the better of her.

We all sat down, had a beautiful meal and chatted away. Eventually, I took my medal collection from my bag and showed them to Lindsey. 'They're great,' she enthused, before heading upstairs. I sat talking to her parents, Janet and Al, until Lindsey returned and dropped two armfuls of medals of all shapes and sizes onto the table. 'What's that one for?' I asked, picking it up. '400 metres individual medley,' she replied. I was stunned. Here was I trying to tell her how good she could become if she put her mind to it, when I would have been better off asking her for a few pointers!

When I asked her for her recorded times over various events, I worked out that, on a not-so-good day for Lindsey and a pretty-good day for me, I might have an outside chance against her in the 50 metres freestyle! I wasn't sure if I should be embarrassed or delighted. In the end I was both. I was delighted to have discovered there was someone else who approached training in the same way as I did, being wary of hypos and constantly trying to prevent them from happening ... but Lindsey's success in swimming went far beyond anything I had achieved. You just had to be there!

13

Nobody told the bumblebee ...

I check my blood sugar levels regularly and consistently, which is very useful when it comes to detecting 'unfelt' hypos. Yes, 'unfelt' hypos. They exist. Really. Sometimes we can be in a state of hypo without realising it, and the only way we can know is via the reading on our glucometers. We can feel perfectly OK, have coherent, intelligent conversations, appear quite unaffected, but sometimes there is a need to eat. I still experience the 'classic' symptoms and **know** I am becoming hypo most times when it happens. Yet there have been times when I have been registering 'Lo' on my glucometer but still felt absolutely fine.

It is another reason that I test myself so often, even though I usually have a good idea where my blood sugars are on the scale. There is an advantage to not feeling hypoglycaemic. If I check myself and I am low, yet feeling all right, I am then in a position to be able to treat the hypo myself, with all my faculties functioning perfectly, without having to be helped. I can even 'enjoy' the treatment of such a hypo.

During hypos, when the symptoms are too strongly felt, we often swallow masses of 'goodies' without really tasting any of them. They are eaten for fuel, not for taste. However, if low and well aware of the fact – but still in control – we are able to eat and savour the 'forbidden fruits', which are not forbidden at this time, without feeling in the least guilty.

For those of us with diabetes, mealtimes are more than simply food preparation and consumption – they can often mean working out maths equations! What do I mean? Many of us when we are due to eat will take an injection. To know how much insulin to take we might check our blood sugar levels and then inject according to the result. However, we may be planning to do something strenuous later on, or perhaps we have already done something, so this is an extra factor that must be added in.

In addition, we have to consider the carbohydrate content of the food – how many grams of this and that? If I want more of it, how much insulin should I take? I'm not particularly hungry – by how many units will I reduce my insulin? Hang on, what was my blood sugar level again? And what was I doing before dinner? What about dessert?

There are lots of things that can influence what we eat and how much insulin to take with it. I am lucky, in a sense, to have had the condition so long that I can usually gauge, with a fair degree of accuracy, the amount of food I will eat and how much insulin to inject to go with it, taking into account my blood sugar level and my previous or forthcoming activities. This comes from personal experience gleaned over many years.

Diabetes is not an exact science and is individual to each of us. It is up to each person with diabetes to find out what is suitable for them. I tested and recorded a lot – and still do. And while it may be inconvenient, or may take some time, I have found it worth doing.

Training without eating extra requires a bit of thought. I tried various experiments, took note of them and learned. After a while, I became used to the amount of insulin and/or food to take, when to take it and the sort of effect it would have on me. I discovered that I needed a certain amount of insulin when I trained so that my blood sugars would not rise. I found out, too, that just because I had a small amount of insulin within me, I would not always become hypo from training. My sugars do not **always** drop down just because I inject a unit or two before training, if they were already up to begin with. So, my fear of hypos has diminished over time, but my awareness that one **could** occur has not. I have also found out how to get away without eating if I do not want to eat and how to eat lots more than is 'recommended' if the fancy takes me.

These discoveries have been made through trial and error, backed by the knowledge of years of living with this condition. If you do decide to try out anything, please **err on the side of caution**. I did. I made mistakes, and, then, if my bloods went up too much I compensated by taking an extra injection. I always had something on hand to eat or drink in case I became hypo. I found these self-experiments well worth the effort. As a result **I** have a much greater understanding of **my** diabetes. **I** am the one living with the condition 24/7. **I** am the one who benefits. **I** also have a much better grip on it. And **I** am most definitely the one who 'controls' it, rather than vice versa.

Many of my discoveries were made during our Four Peaks Challenge training. Ever since I became involved with the Four Peaks I have enjoyed the hills and mountains. Not only have I seen some spectacular scenery and experienced a huge array of emotions, I have also come to appreciate the effects that hillwalking can have on a person with diabetes.

A walk usually takes the best part of a day, including travelling. Hillwalking is a continuous exercise, lasting for many hours. When we were training for the Four Peaks I found that even with a cut in insulin my bloods tended to drop after we had had lunch, because we had walked for many hours before lunch. Hillwalking, however, can be done at a pace where eating en route is feasible. I can eat away happily as we walk along, knowing that my blood sugar level is maintained at a happy, healthy position.

When you eat while walking it does not cause nausea or cramping, as it is likely to do when you swim or run as a form of exercise. Nor does it cause you to need the toilet in a hurry! We also discovered that after a day's walking we needed more carbohydrates than usual later that evening and often a cut in our night-time insulin dose, such was the impact of continuous exercise through the day.

Hillwalking has a number of advantages for those of us with diabetes. It allows us to eat more tasty 'junk' food. It usually requires us to reduce our insulin intake both before and after the walk, while at the same time enjoying extra food. The views can be amazing and it is a great way to spend a day. What better incentives could there be?

When we did the Four Peaks Challenge most of us were involved to prove to the rest of the world what we already knew – that people with diabetes were in just as good, if not better, condition than anyone else. We wanted to bury a variety of myths and misconceptions and to demonstrate that people with diabetes can and will perform tasks set for them. We also wanted to show other people with diabetes that if we could do this, so could you!

A couple of months after the Four Peaks Challenge, the Wicklow Mountain Rescue Team organised a fund-raising night hike. After all their help during our adventure, we felt we should repay them by taking part in this event. A few of our Challenge team got together with a navigator, Brian Byrne, who also had had diabetes for 30 years. He became our mentor and adviser during our training that summer. We also invited two other young people with diabetes: Robbie, my cousin, and Celine, whom we had met at the Irish Diabetic Association's (IDA) AGM a few weeks earlier and who had never climbed a mountain before. What an introduction!

Seven of us met at the foot of Lughnaquilla at 4 p.m. on a wet, cold, breezy December evening. We were a varied group of individuals with one uniting factor – we all had diabetes. We started climbing into the all-enveloping gloom and before long had to switch on our torches in order to make headway. Without them, visibility was nil. There was also a howling gale and almost horizontal rain. This was the sort of night for wrapping up warm and snug in front of a blazing fire. However, we were out in the elements, being lashed by wind and rain ... and having the time of our lives!

At one point, we all switched off our torches and stood, still and silent, so that the experience of being out there in the wild, with no artificial light, could be experienced. I found it both

thrilling and terrifying. Then the inevitable happened –
someone started to do a blood test in the raging weather
conditions and the dark. We formed a circle round whoever
was performing the test, one person holding a torch, the rest
trying to keep the rain off. This was a real group effort taking,
in rotation, the role of torch-bearer, provider of shelter and
tester.

We continued up and on until we reached the top of the
mountain, where we stopped for some well-earned soup and
sandwiches. Just before we ate, we all checked our bloods
again. I wonder what sort of sight we made – seven of us
sitting on the top of a mountain in the dark of a miserable,
wet and windy December night, each of us with a pinprick of
blood on the tips of our fingers. There has to be an *X-Files*
story there somewhere!!

The blood sugar readings generally ranged from 3 to 13
except for Celine, for whom this was a first-time experience.
She had a perfect reading of 7. It just shows what people with
diabetes can do with a bit of support and some self-confidence.
It is also a good example of people with diabetes being able to
do whatever it is they set out to do.

Around 11 p.m. we boarded the bus and were taken off to a
local pub where we spent several hours, revelling in a
wonderful atmosphere, until at 2 a.m. we headed home to
bed, tired but very happy.

During our training for the Four Peaks Challenge, Brian
was with us as a hillwalking mentor and as a diabetic adviser.
He is an extremely fit person, fitter than most people, whether
they have diabetes or not. A few years after he was diagnosed,
he wanted to enter a marathon. He went to his doctor for some
advice about training, insulin intake and so on, so that he could
prepare properly and participate at the highest level. 'The
marathon?' said his incredulous doctor. 'You cannot do the
marathon. **Diabetics cannot do that sort of thing**.' 'But
I did it last year,' Brian pointed out.

How **dare** anyone say anything like that about those of us
with diabetes. Brian's reply spoke volumes. He had already
completed a marathon before, without much help or advice
from anyone, as far as his diabetes was concerned. Is it any

wonder that it is hard to listen to anyone, a doctor or not, who says something you know not to be true? How can we be expected to trust people and adhere to their advice if we don't trust this advice or feel we know more than they do, which can often be the case?

According to recognised aerodynamic tests, the bumblebee cannot fly because of the shape and weight of its body in relation to the total wing area. But the bumblebee doesn't know this, so he goes ahead and flies anyway ... I cannot begin to tell you the number of times I have been told that having diabetes means that I 'cannot have sugar' or I 'cannot drink alcohol' or even that I 'have to eat lots of sugar'.

There are times when it is highly inadvisable to eat sugar, but there are also times when it is exactly what people with diabetes should do. As for alcohol, I do not drink it – my own choice – but I have been out with people with diabetes who have drunk as much as anyone else in the company – and it had the same effect on them – a hangover! What is irritating is when people with diabetes are authoritatively told what we 'can' and 'cannot' do by people who do not really know what on earth they are talking about.

I am not saying people with diabetes should go out and drink. That has to be each person's own decision, just as it is mine not to. But no one knows the effects of alcohol on them until they try it. People with diabetes have to get to know their own limitations and understand the effect alcohol will have if they choose to indulge, just like everyone else.

I have been told that I would not survive if I missed a meal, or that I could not be a safe driver, just because I have diabetes. How wrong can people be? I have spent so much of my life involved in sport and training that it is impossible to calculate just how far I have walked or run and how many metres I have swum. All of this activity has placed physical demands on my body, demands which a lot of medics would have thought too much for a person with diabetes.

People with diabetes are told that they have to pay extra on insurance premiums that cover them to drive as they are 'high risk'. In some cases people with diabetes are not allowed to drive at all. I learned to drive in 1992 and have been driving on and off ever since. I never drive unless I check my blood sugar levels before sitting behind the wheel. Even when it was perfectly safe for me to drive, I would not go anywhere without taking a bottle of Lucozade **and** a bar of chocolate with me.

I am ultra-cautious, but I still have diabetes. Therefore, I am considered to be 'high risk'. Yet Ireland and the UK still allow people with alcohol in their systems to drive. How many accidents and deaths are due to drivers being under the influence of alcohol? Drivers who drink are still legally permitted to have a certain amount of alcohol in their system when they drive. Why don't statisticians record just how often people with diabetes get safely from A to B? It would be too boring, that's why, because it happens time and time again.

Surely insurance assessments should be done on an individual basis, assessing each driver with diabetes? Diabetes **is** a consideration when driving, I wholly agree. However, we are more likely to be safer drivers because we are more likely to know what sort of physical state we are in before we get into the car, through checking our blood sugar levels. We deserve to be assessed on our own merits, rather than all be categorised as 'high risk'.

People with diabetes always have trouble getting insured. Whenever I have taken out a policy with an insurance company, I have always had to fill in details about my diabetes. How long have I had it? Have I got Type 1 or Type 2? And the one that baffles me: how many units of insulin do I take daily? What a ridiculous question! I can understand insurance companies wanting to know if we are in good health and if our diabetes is an extra risk, but to ask how many units of insulin a day we take really takes the biscuit.

What difference does it make? Some days I will take 42 units, on another day I will take 32 and on another 60 units. Why? Because I know how to control my diabetes and I know that different situations call for different measures. What does it matter how many units of insulin is taken if we are in charge of our diabetes and have it under control?

Insurance companies should treat us as individuals and ask our doctors how much of a risk we are. We are all different people leading different sorts of lifestyles and taking different

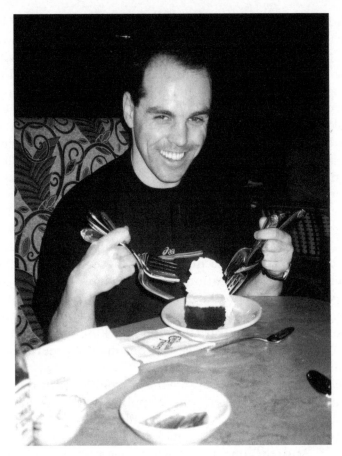

Figure 10   John – in Providence, Rhode Island –
'Doing something I "shouldn't" ...'.

amounts of insulin. We **deserve** to be treated individually. Take into account our **individual** general health, our **individual** grasp of our condition and the **individual** lifestyles we lead. It is just not fair to say we are **all** high-risk people.

For the record, after we had climbed up and down Lughnaquilla that stormy December night, Brian and I drove from the south of Wicklow to Dublin without any trouble at all. In fact, we stopped to help a driver who had run off the road and helped him push his car so that he could get home.

People with diabetes who drive are just as capable as anyone else of being safe drivers.

Diabetes **can** be controlled. Through trial and error and experience, we can control it. It might still have a bearing on how I prepare for something, or influence what I might or might not consume, but it is **not** the supreme authority that rules my life. It is not the only thing I consider when I decide to try something new. I make diabetes fit into my lifestyle, rather than submitting to its demands. I do not let it stop me from enjoying my life, nor do I ignore it. I do however **control** it.

I have heard many times in the past, from my doctors, that they were going to 'try something to see if it works.' Surely that is a trial-and-error approach? From errors we can learn how to avoid a recurrence of a particular problem. If a dose of insulin is not sufficient to keep my blood sugars down where I want them to be, for example, I will know the next time I am in a similar situation to increase the dose.

Making mistakes is not absolutely necessary in order to learn, but doing so is human. We all make mistakes. They are not our only teachers, but they **can** teach us if we let them – even if the lesson is sometimes a hard one. At some stage or other, no matter how experienced we are, we may be in a situation we have never been in before and that brings the possibility of making a mistake.

I would urge everyone not to let fear of making mistakes stop you from trying anything. I have learned from all my mistakes over the years. You can learn from yours. Go on, try something. You could make a lot of valuable self-discoveries in the process. **BUT DO NOT BE RECKLESS!** Approach whatever you are going to do with caution and care, but carry on with it. Diabetes can only stop us if we let it, so **DO NOT LET IT!**

Tips and hints

Hypoglycaemia

People with diabetes are advised to keep their blood glucose levels as near to the normal blood glucose levels as possible. Normal blood glucose levels in non-diabetic people range between 4 and 7 mmol/l. If blood glucose levels drop below normal, whatever the cause, this is called hypoglycaemia (a hypo). It is important that even mild hypos – or lows – which can be easily treated by the intake of a sugary drink or food, are reported to your doctor.

Some golden rules:

- always have some form of quickly absorbed glucose with you;
- never drive with a hypo – if warning signs come on while driving, always stop the car and get into the passenger seat, so you are not seen to be in control of a vehicle while hypoglycaemic;
- when driving, always keep glucose or sweets in an accessible place – the glove compartment is not always very accessible;
- stop every so often when driving, to check blood sugar levels;
- if you are a carer and unable to treat an unconscious hypo, call the emergency services or your GP;
- if the hypo is accompanied by vomiting, drowsiness and difficulty breathing, a doctor is needed and the person should be admitted to hospital.

14

Everything's alright ...

At one of the Diabetes Federation of Ireland's (DFI) AGMs, the editor of *Identity*, the DFI magazine, announced her resignation. It was then said that if anyone was interested in taking on the role of editor, the DFI would love to hear from them. I was sitting at the back of the auditorium, and it was as if everyone suddenly turned round and looked at me expectantly! I had written various articles for *Identity*, on the Four Peaks Challenge and about the first children's camp. I had also had a letter published in the magazine. This led to a general air of expectancy that I would become editor of *Identity*.

So, I took on the job at the beginning of 2000. It represented a chance to meet a lot more people with diabetes, and I also felt that the magazine could be used as a vehicle for helping more people to meet each other. I found it tough-going at times. I was also working full-time in my 'real' job, as well as trying to keep fit and finish the counselling skills course. Most of my work on *Identity* took place after I had finished 'work', but even though it was tough I enjoyed my involvement with it. It also gave me opportunities that I would never have otherwise had. One day I received an email from the DFI, informing me of a World Meeting of the International

Committee of Diabetes Magazines, to be held in Cuernavaca, Mexico, in November 2000.

My initial reaction was that I did not want to go. The truth was that I was terrified! I would have to travel to Mexico – alone – and my heart thumped at the thought of everything that could go wrong. However, I did agree to go and arrangements were made for my travel and accommodation.

On 1 November I boarded the flight bound for Newark, New Jersey, to make a connecting flight that would take me to Mexico. For the first time in my life I had to cope with a 36-hour day from a diabetic perspective. I was travelling through time zones, which I had never done before, and I wasn't too sure how this would affect me. Added to that was the natural tension, which had been messing around with my blood sugars, but once I got going I had no choice but to cope.

I kept checking my blood sugars and for the whole trip to the United States they were constantly in the teen numbers. This was probably because of the extra adrenaline from being nervous, but more likely because I kept eating whatever food they put in front of me on the plane. I had no desire to become hypo, and I was making very sure that this would not happen.

About an hour away from arrival in Mexico, I slumped in my window seat, dozing uncomfortably, when I woke to a song, piped through the headphones, which I recognised from a musical. I had been to see the show a year ago and had loved it. It was not just the music that made it for me – the subject matter also held a lot of meaning for me. *Everything's Alright* from *Jesus Christ Superstar* was coming through the headphones. The lines I heard were:

> Try not to get worried, try not to turn on to
> Problems that upset you, oh don't you know
> Everything's alright, yes, everything's fine
> And we want you to sleep well tonight . . .

The relief I felt was incredible! It was as if the words were directed straight at me. As I flicked through the in-flight

magazine, however, I found the listings page for each channel –
Everything's Alright was not on any play list!

The customs area in Mexico was a great big buzz of
activity – all in Spanish – not a single word of which
I understood. I had visited the Mexican Embassy in Dublin
before I left to ask for a card I could carry. The card stated in
Spanish that I had diabetes and that I was carrying insulin and
injections. This was in case I was quizzed in customs or if
something happened to me.

I had to make my way back to the airport the following day,
as this was the pre-arranged rendezvous point from where
editors of diabetes magazines from around the world would
be collected and taken to Cuernavaca, about an hour's drive
south of Mexico City.

The International Diabetes Federation was organising the
event, and one of their staff was Irish, from Dublin. So, I had
some contact I felt I could turn to in case of a crisis.

At the beginning of the meeting, each delegate's first task
was to present their magazines to the others. I sat in the
audience, as the first speaker got up and presented his
country's magazine ... as did the next speaker ... and the
next. Only then did I catch on that I was going to be asked
to talk about *Identity*, and I hadn't got a single thing prepared.
I had completely overlooked the fact that everyone had been
asked to do a presentation. I quickly grabbed a pen, made a few
notes and waited until it was my turn to speak.

The official language of the meeting was English, which
was obviously not a problem for me, but neither did it seem
to be a problem for any of the other delegates, no matter from
where in the world they came. I was soon called and went up to
the front of the auditorium. 'Being Irish,' I began. 'I have a
habit of speaking too quickly, so if I am going too fast, please
don't be afraid to tell me to shut up!' There was an immediate
burst of laughter and I started to relax. 'They are on my side,'
I thought.

I spoke about who I was, what the DFI was, where we
were – geographically and concerning other aspects – and
about the problems I faced as editor of *Identity*. 'How did
I do that?' I mused, as I returned to my seat.

After the presentations we had dinner and I got the chance to mix and chat with the others. Soon, I made one of those amazing 'small world' discoveries: the editor of the South African magazine *Diabetes Focus*, Susan Leuner, was a masters swimmer – and she knew one of the swimmers whom I have seen regularly at the galas in Ireland.

I discovered something else – most of the editors from the other diabetes magazines were either professional journalists, who worked full-time on their magazines, or extremely dedicated health care professionals. I was one of only two editors who actually **had** diabetes, the other was the editor from Turkey. I found this out when he asked me if he could have some of my insulin as his had got lost en route to Mexico.

Over the weekend meeting, I went to a variety of workshops. By now I had really settled into my role as a participant in this worldwide event, and at the final group session I was asked to be the chair. It showed delegates had confidence in me, which in turn did wonders for my own self-confidence.

Before I left Ireland, I had not been keen on travelling across the world alone to spend time with a group of strangers. However, I thoroughly enjoyed my experience with such remarkable people from all corners of the earth. I flew home feeling much happier for having made the trip. I had learned a lot while I was there, which would help me in editing *Identity* and I had also gained experience in travelling through time zones with my diabetes.

In July 2001 I managed to compete in the European Masters Swimming Championships (EMSC) in Palma, Majorca, for my club, Aer Lingus Masters. I competed in three races and two relays. I swam in the 50 metres freestyle, breaststroke and backstroke events and in the mixed medley (two men and two women) relay and the mixed freestyle relay.

We finished 47th out of 52 in the 4×50 metres mixed medley relay and 50th out of 58 teams in the 4×50 metres mixed freestyle relay, both in the 120+ years category (i.e., the combined age of the four swimmers in the team). I was not going to let my diabetes hold me back, and while we were

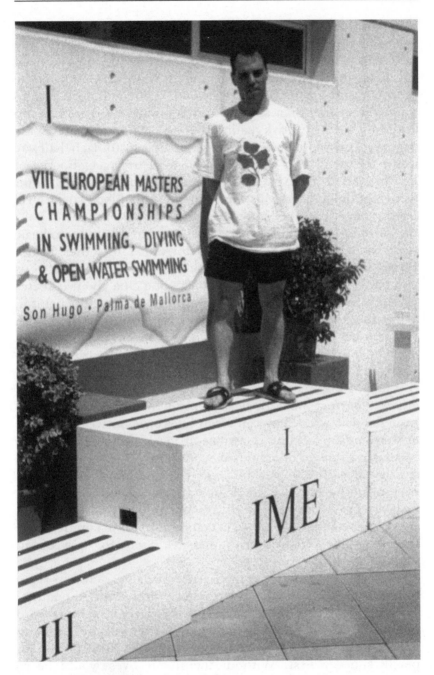

Figure 11   John – 'I wish!' – EMSC, July 2001.

way down the rankings I had gone to take part and give my all, swimming progressively faster in each race.

On one of the days I did not even bother to eat from breakfast until late in the evening. I was swimming in the morning and again in the afternoon. The swimmers had to be at the calling area about 30 minutes before their race, so I didn't want to risk eating before swimming, with the probable consequence of having an upset stomach halfway down the pool! Nor did I want to miss my race. Food just had to wait. I got by doing a blood test and injecting a unit or two of quick-acting insulin to prevent my blood sugar level from rising. It worked a treat.

Through all my life with diabetes, I have found two basic types of medic. One is the doctor/nurse or other health professional who thinks they know it all and who talks to us in a patronising way, as if we hadn't got a clue about diabetes and its effects. The other type is the pleasant, friendly, helpful, sympathetic, hard-working doctor/nurse or other health professional who on top of their hectic working hours can often be found volunteering their time, knowledge, profession-alism and so on to help people with diabetes.

Since I became involved with the DFI, I have often been amazed at just how dedicated some of these health care professionals are. They can often be seen – on weeknights or at weekends – tackling questions at local meetings. They are regularly involved in organising committees for various events associated with diabetes and attend kids camps, information evenings, Sweetpea Kidz Clubs (more on this later) in a professional – but almost always unpaid – capacity, so that the event can go ahead. We could not, for example, have taken 20-plus children with diabetes away for a weekend without medical back-up.

To me, this highlights their sense of dedication to serving others, their willingness to help others without any thought of reward. They rarely get any reward, except maybe a word of thanks, which is often immediately followed by a plea to come back again! It is all done because they put other people's needs first. Without them, our lives would be so much more difficult.

Diabetes-wise, 2001 was a very rewarding year for me. This was the year I got involved with the DFI's Sweetpea Kidz Club, run by Mairead Fanning, a schoolteacher who has had diabetes even longer than I. This club was set up for families of children with diabetes, and in April I went on my first weekend away with them to Trabolgan in Cork.

The weekend was for parents to share experiences about what it is like to have a child with diabetes and the impact it can have on every single member of the family. I went along to help and offer a bit of support to the parents and to the kids themselves. It was good to be asked to get involved with this, as I could share my experiences of having been a child with diabetes. Maybe this could help the parents to understand the sorts of feelings and emotions a diabetic child can face.

It was also the year in which the DFI, in conjunction with Diabetes UK (Northern Ireland) held its own first all-Ireland Youth Conference at the Delphi Activity Centre in County Mayo in October. A mix of young Irish adults from all parts of this island, all with diabetes, shared – some for the first time ever – their own experiences and feelings of how life with diabetes was for them.

I was thrilled that this event had been set up. Over five years earlier I had stood at an airport, almost in tears, unhappy at leaving behind all my new and understanding friends as I left to go home to a lack of support for the emotional and psychological side of my diabetic life. Yet, through hoping, praying, participating, plaguing and lobbying the right people, it had now come to pass.

Feedback was extremely positive. The only complaint I heard was that it did not last long enough. It was so good to see people who had come to the weekend expressing themselves and their feelings about their lives with diabetes. Problems were brought out and aired and made easier to deal with, myths and lies were banished and many more friendships were formed. At last a new way of thinking about diabetes had come to Ireland.

It had meant so much to me to see people becoming more well informed about their diabetes. I know that most of those who were there went away feeling much more positive about their life, and many expressed their gratitude. Control was now firmly in their hands, which was where it should be. Young people with diabetes in Ireland now had a much stronger voice than they had ever had before ... at long last!

15

Parting shots

How long before a cure is found? That is the question we all want answered. Even so, it cannot be answered with any certainty. Diabetes has been around for thousands of years, but it was not until 1922 that the first life-saving insulin injection was given. Prior to the discovery of insulin, the only treatment for diabetes was ... starvation. What a choice to have to make: would you prefer to die from the condition or from the treatment? In other words, diabetes was a killer.

Note I say 'was'. Thank goodness it is different nowadays. Having diabetes does not necessarily mean an untimely demise. It has its trials, as we know, but it is treatable and can be lived with. Even so, we still want to know when a cure will be found.

Anything is possible, of course, and research into diabetes is always taking place throughout the world, but so far no cure has been discovered. Many findings have been made: different types of insulin have been manufactured, blood-testing machines have been developed and are freely available and in rare cases pancreatic transplants have taken place. Yet it seems to me that it will be a long time into the future before a cure will be found. I just feel that this condition has a while to go yet before we get rid of it.

If a cure is discovered, it will come as a great relief to many people. Yet I feel that those of us who have had diabetes for most of our lives, for whom it has become a large part of our lifestyles, will take some time to adjust to a world free of injections and blood tests and to a world where we don't have to watch what we eat and drink.

It would have an enormous effect on me if I did not have to prepare my meal to go with my activities. If I did not have to check my blood sugar levels before a training session. If I did not have to make a calculation of everything I was about to eat. I suppose that in some ways I could be seen as having become rather 'institutionalised'.

If cured of diabetes, would we go on a chocolate binge for days on end? Would we have plates piled high with chips, biscuits, cakes, sandwiches and sweets and choose a bigger dessert than our main meal? How drunk would we become in our rapture? I reckon if you asked anyone with Type 1 diabetes what they would do if they were cured out of the blue, most would answer that they would 'pig out' on chocolate. Fair enough, I would probably do the same. But where would we draw the line?

I do feel this could be a real issue for those of us with diabetes. Potentially, we could go from being perfectly healthy people with a certain condition, to being overfed and overweight with a wealth of problems stored up for the future including obesity, high cholesterol levels and heart disease from overeating unbalanced, unhealthy diets and lack of exercise. I feel that it would take time to adjust to a life without diabetes.

Insulin pumps seem to be gaining popularity in the treatment of diabetes, with more medical companies producing them. These pumps provide a continuous supply of insulin which is automatically delivered to the recipient and boosted at mealtimes by a manually selected amount to suit each individual's needs. Pumps consist of an insulin reservoir, which is bigger than a regular syringe, a small battery-operated pump and a computer chip that allows the user to control exactly how much insulin is to be delivered via the pump.

The insulin is delivered to the body through a thin plastic tube or *infusion set* and consists of a needle or *cannula*, which is soft. This is inserted under the skin, usually on the abdomen, and is changed every two to three days. The pump delivers insulin to the body 24 hours a day, according to a programmed plan made unique to each wearer. A small amount of insulin is delivered on an ongoing basis – the **basal** or long-acting dose – and when food is eaten the pump is programmed to deliver a **bolus**, or quick-acting dose, to match the amount of food to be consumed. It is up to the user of the pump to decide on the amount of insulin to be given.

On a personal level, the idea of a pump constantly attached to my body holds no appeal whatsoever. I have found that anyone who uses a pump seems to love it, but many with whom I have discussed the idea and who do not want to wear one say the same as me: 'No thanks!' I am happy to rely on my multi-injection regime. On the other hand, lots of people have gained more satisfaction from wearing a pump. At least we now have a choice. It is up to the person with diabetes to decide whether she or he is happier with or without a pump.

Another question we have all asked is: why not perform pancreas transplants on people with diabetes, so that we can produce our own insulin and not have to rely on injections? It seems obvious to those of us with diabetes and a reasonable question to ask.

Pancreas transplants have taken place usually, however, when the person with diabetes is undergoing a transplant of another organ, such as a liver or more commonly a kidney. This is because the treatment that is needed to prevent the organ recipient from rejecting the donor organ(s) can cause more damage to the body than treating their diabetes with insulin.

Immunosuppressant drugs must be taken for the rest of the transplant recipient's life. These drugs have side effects that can include developing skin and/or cervical cancer. There is also a great risk of infection, because the immunosuppressants reduce the body's defence mechanisms. There is also a lack of available organs. Organs for transplant are obtained from accident victims. Because of this there will never be enough pancreases available for transplantation.

For some reason, a lot of people with diabetes seem reluctant to join their diabetes association. Why is this? Perhaps some people do not want anyone to know about their diabetes or do not want to talk about it. Fair enough, that is their decision and quite understandable. But the more people who join their diabetes association the stronger it will become, with more people available to offer and provide help, or to start things happening.

There will be a larger pool of ideas, experience and knowledge to be called on. Having a large diabetes association gives that organisation a louder, stronger voice, especially when it comes to lobbying for funding, or trying to effect changes in attitudes, or mobilising opposition to insurance companies who continue to discriminate. It is easier to stand with many when it comes to fighting your corner than it is to stand with just a few. If you are not already a member, why not join your association? It can only be to your benefit.

Before I joined what is now the Diabetes Federation of Ireland (DFI), I knew far fewer people in the same boat as me. I had diabetes for a long time before I realised that I needed help, someone to talk to who understood. Joining my association has opened many doors for me, doors which might have remained closed, imprisoning me in a world where I was the only one who understood my situation.

I got a great deal out of my first Youth Diabetic (YD) weekend experience and have continued to get a lot out of belonging to an organisation ever since. I also try to put something back whenever I can. I was taught how to facilitate groups, I have learned counselling skills, I was lucky enough to go on various children's camps as a leader – experiences which I have found to be most enriching. By getting involved I have gained so much, without even having to look much further than the associations. I have thoroughly enjoyed all of these benefits and experiences. If you do decide to join, it does not mean you have committed yourself for life – you are free to leave at any stage. But really, what have you got to lose by joining?

Having diabetes has actually given me opportunities to do things and meet people that I might not have had the chance to do if I did not have the condition. My circle of friends has increased through involvement in a variety of activities, and I have met some truly brilliant people – all because I have diabetes. Of course, it is not the only thing we have in common – friendship goes much deeper than that and diabetes is not our only topic of conversation – but it did serve to bring us together.

People who see diabetes youth conferences advertised automatically assume that **all** we talk about is diabetes. We do discuss it, sometimes at length and in great detail, but when we spend weekends away with each other we also talk about lots of other things: football, work, college, holidays, books, which is funnier – the *X-Files* or *Due South?*, why Freddie Mercury was the best singer **ever**, why Homer Simpson is **king** of television ... the list could go on and on.

How often have you wondered why **you** happen to be the only one you know to have been burdened with this horrible condition? I have wondered, and not just once or twice. However, when I take a step back and have a look at the impact it has had on my life, I think I may have found an answer as to why **I** got it.

I was diagnosed at a very young age. I have no memory of life without diabetes. I have had over 27,000 injections in my life. I went through a lot – fear, worry, lack of self-confidence, I felt I was an imposition on others – all negative feelings. I became timid and fearful a lot of the time. In short, it caused me suffering, which I can still recall.

By feeling this suffering, I have found it easier to relate to anyone who has ever turned to me for help or advice. If I had not experienced all the fear, pain and even the guilt which came with having diabetes, I do not think I would be able to imagine the feelings and emotions felt by others who live with the condition.

I believe my sometimes frightening and often painful memories are the key to my understanding what others have gone through and are going through. I like to think that I was 'given' diabetes so that I could try to help others to come to terms with it. This may sound rather self-absorbed, possibly even arrogant, which I hope is not the case, but it makes sense to me.

I have begun to see my diabetes as a gift. My outlook for too long was: because of diabetes I **cannot** do ... Now I ask myself: what **can** I do with this? My going to the children's camps came about through having the same condition as the kids. I go to help – but I have to admit that I often feel more of a participant than a leader or adviser. It's not often that you get to jump into the sea from the edge of a pier under the guise of learning-by-doing, or to see extremely talented kids perform on stage – for free.

All the pains, the jabs and the worries brought about by diabetes have been transformed into joy, laughter, sharing, loving and watching people grow and develop. These far outweigh any of the negative aspects diabetes has brought into my life.

Earlier on, I asked the question I'm sure we have all asked ourselves: why me? Now, after all of the advances I have made with my diabetes, I look at myself and ask: why not me? Yes, I have had my share of problems – the unmerciful hypos, the years of guilt and fear, the constant pressure to be 'in control' and to 'get it right'. But I have learned to deal with it and live with it.

I suppose in some ways it is like a relationship – some good days, some not so good. But, all the same, I still have to live with it, so I might as well do my best to get on with it. As a result of looking at it in a different light, I have turned diabetes into a positive influence in my life.

It has taught me the value of listening to and looking after my body, not just in a diabetic sense. It has encouraged me to be aware of living and enjoying my life, rather than enduring it or letting it pass me by. Possibly, it has taught me to be a good listener too.

My own, very personal opinion is that God gave me diabetes to see what I could do with it. For years it was a burden, a curse and I suffered in untold and unseen ways.

However, through that suffering, I know what it is like to go through what others go through, those people who ask for advice or who just want to talk to someone about it.

Diabetes was my teacher and has prepared me for the next stage in my personal development. Having come out of the dark tunnel, where I meandered aimlessly for too long, I now feel strong enough to go on with diabetes in my life, possibly even strong enough to try to help others who may need help. What is the point of my having all of these years of experience, if I do not use them to help someone else? Once knowledge is gained it is not lost if shared, if anything it grows. By giving it away we lose none of it, so why keep it to ourselves?

I feel that I have diabetes for a reason, that reason being to go and help others who have it. I know it seems a bit airy-fairy and it may seem totally strange to many people, but I genuinely do believe this to be the case. Through living most of my life with it, I have encountered the problems, the prejudices and the fears that living with it brings. I went through the works: trying to face up to the fact that, based on today's knowledge, I will be injecting myself with insulin for the rest of my life; the hypos; hypers; fear; feeling different; anxieties when trying something new; not being understood; lack of sympathy; guilt – at something that was not my fault in any way. I think that I can offer myself to someone who wants to have a 'bitch' about life, who needs a shoulder to cry on or who wants to share laughter at some of what we come across. I feel that diabetes was my signpost in life to show me where to go, what to do and even whom to meet.

For ages I thought of diabetes as a curse. I thought this for years. However, when I recall what I have done in my life and the people I have met, I realise that a lot of the good things in my life were a direct result of my having diabetes. I have met great people, experienced events that will live in my memory until I die, discovered a bit of a writer within me and, in doing so, I have shown myself that I can do whatever I put my mind to doing.

I now see diabetes as being **my** gift from God, **my** gateway to the paths I have taken and will take in the future, instead of a closed door, barring my progress. Also, because I feel so strongly about those people whom I have met directly through my diabetes, if I was told I could go back and relive my life over again, free of diabetes, but that it would mean losing all contacts and friends I have met through having the condition, I would opt to keep diabetes in my life, because I love my friends.

I would not be offended, though, if one of my friends who has diabetes chose to live their life again free of diabetes ... but sacrificed their friendship with me, meaning we would never meet again. That is fine. I would still like to have that person in my life, but I would totally understand someone wanting to be free of their diabetes. I see my diabetes as having led me to great things and, more importantly, to exceptional, wonderful people who are gifted and extraordinary and whom I love. Even with all the negativity that goes with having diabetes, I am grateful for being a person with diabetes.

One day, a few years back, during our Four Peaks Challenge training, a discussion began about whether we were *diabetics* or *people with diabetes*. At the time, it was something to which I had never given much thought. I had always said that I was *a diabetic* or even that I was *diabetic*, something I must have picked up from when I was first diagnosed. During this discussion, it was suggested that being referred to as *a diabetic* was a labelling term and it made me look back to articles written before the 1990s which used the term *diabetic* more often than not when referring to people with the condition. *Diabetes* is used too, of course, but usually in reference to the condition, whereas *diabetic* tended to refer to the person with diabetes.

With political correctness, we were later more likely to be referred to as being *a person/people with diabetes*. The DFI had changed its name from the Irish Diabetic Association. The British Diabetic Association (BDA) is now Diabetes UK. I think these changes have had an influence on the terminology now in common use.

On reflection, I tend to favour the term *people with diabetes* as it recognises us as people who have a condition, rather than the word *diabetic* which puts the condition first and the person second. But, to be perfectly honest, I do not mind which term

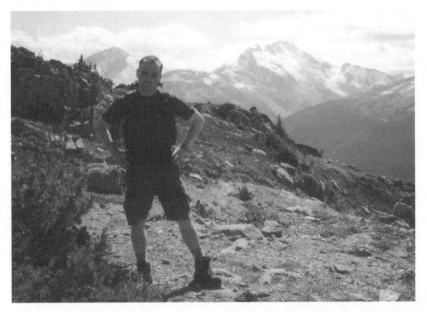

Figure 12   Whistler Mountain, Canada, September 2001.

is used in reference to me. I am a person who knows who I am and can speak up for myself. I am well aware of who I am, what I am and how I am. Being *diabetic* or *having diabetes* is not the only part of me – there is a lot more than that. *Diabetic* is a label, it's true, so is *husband, swimmer, reader, Christian, friend, brother, son, writer* – all of which I am, but none of which I find an offensive term.

The bottom line is: I need insulin. How I am referred to after that is the other person's choice!

Appendix: painting by numbers

I wrote the following poem after I had paid a visit to a friend, Kate, whom I had met at one of the Youth Diabetic (YD) weekends over in England.

When we do our blood tests, on certain makes of strips (after the blood has been blotted from the strip before it is put into the glucometer) the strip then turns from being yellow before the blood has been applied to varying shades after the blood has been blotted from it. The darker the colour becomes usually reflects a more elevated blood sugar reading.

I was visiting Kate in her new yet-to-be-decorated house. We were discussing different colours and different shades, and in which rooms the colours would look best.

I don't know which of us brought it up, but the shades were compared with the colours that remain on the strips after the dabbing away of the blood. We began to come out with statements like *The wall over there being a lovely shade of 5.4*, or the living room being imagined as being *A nice shade of 12.7*, or whatever we happened to come up with. It was ridiculous, but we found it hilarious, and later on I managed to compose the following verse which I hope can be appreciated by all, but which I have a feeling will only *fully*

be appreciated, understood and enjoyed by those of us with
diabetes.

So, with apologies to everyone in advance, here
goes . . . :

PAINTING-BY-NUMBERS ... FOR REAL!!!
Entering the front room
Just catching the morning sun
Enhancing the hue and ambience
A nice shade of Five Point One

Upon the floor the carpet
But not to be trod on by shoes
A gentle hint of aqua-marine
Which we call Six Point Two

Further on into the living room
At table we sit after tea
A reflection of our indulgences
'Is that coloured Nineteen Point Three?'

To the immediate left, the kitchen
Fridge freezer with goodies galore
'I was thinking of doing this in
A nice bright Four Point Four ...'

The Hob-Nobs are kept well out of sight
– But they can keep you alive
You may help yourself to them
If you drop below Three Point Five

We haven't left this room yet
Have some Weetabix
Recommended by every known (Knowing? –
Dunno about that ...) dietitian
To maintain a steady Six!!

Back out then, to don your overalls
– Keep those Colours even!
Try a combination of Reds or Greens
– Paint it Nine Point Seven!

Turn around for the bathroom
Showered – then floor quite wet
It darkened this brightness of the room
From Seven to Eleven Point Eight

Finally the bedroom
Painting a new design
'I wonder what would look good here?
– I know: Five Point Nine!'

The paintwork is complete by now
I've told you blow by blow
A whole new meaning to painting by numbers
– But what shade is Six Point Oh?

Will we ever obtain that figurative colour?
Or will everything be green?
(If you don't know what I mean by that
It's a number ending in '-teen'!!)

Our colour code is almost done
What we want is brown
Because the colours so described
Are a contrast between Up and Down!

Another day your sugars may be raised
So we might rearrange the shelves
This should bring your levels right back down
From being way Up at Twelve!!

(John Keeler, 20 June 1999)

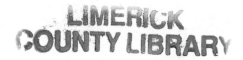

Glossary

Actrapid A quick-acting insulin. Theoretically, it should be injected 30–40 minutes before a meal. It lasts between 6 and 7 hours (on average) in a person's system and usually requires the person taking this type of insulin to eat in-between meals (John Keeler).

Blood glucose (sugar) level The blood sugar level is measured in *millimoles per litre of blood* (mmol/l). In the non-diabetic it will always be between 4 and 10 mmol/l. We diabetics don't have it that easy!! (John Keeler).

Carbohydrates Any of a large group of energy-producing organic compounds containing carbon, hydrogen and oxygen, e.g., starch, glucose and other sugars (*The Concise Oxford Dictionary*, 9th edn).

This is what helps us to stop or prevent us from going hypo (John Keeler).

Diabetes A condition caused by a deficiency in the production of insulin by the body. Sugar and starch are not properly metabolized and the blood and uring contain excessive amounts of sugars, causing risk of convulsions and coma (*The Concise Oxford Dictionary*, 9th edn).

A lifetime of injections, blood tests, hospital visits, hypos, hypers and a whole lot more – see inside! Also known as *insulin-dependent diabetes mellitus* (IDDM) or *Type 1 diabetes* (as opposed to Type 2 diabetes, barely even mentioned in here, as I am Type 1) (John Keeler).

Glucometer   The machines we use to measure our own blood sugar/glucose levels. In Ireland and the UK, it is measures by millimoles per litre of blood (mmol/l) and 'ideally' should be between 4 and 10. Anything below 4 is considered 'low' or 'hypoglycaemic', anything above 10 is considered to be 'hyperglycaemic'. In other countries, it is measured by milligrammes per litre of blood (mg/l). The equivalent to mmol/l in mg/l is obtained by multiplying by 18 (i.e., 6 mmol/l is equal to 108 mg/l: $6 \times 18 = 108$) (John Keeler).

HbA1c level   Our 'average' blood glucose level over a period of time. The 'optimum' level for this to be at is 6%. This is what (some) doctors judge our diabetes control by (John Keeler).

Humalog   A much faster-acting insulin. Gets to work after about 10–15 minutes after being injected and has a working lifespan in one's system of about 5–6 hours. Does not always require a person to eat between meals (John Keeler).

Humulin I   A long-acting insulin, with a lifespan of about 12 hours (John Keeler).

Hyperglycaemia   An excess of glucose in the bloodstream (*The Concise Oxford Dictionary*, 9th edn).

When we do not have enough insulin in our system to deal with the amount of carbohydrates or sugars which are present in our systems, hypers (raised blood sugar levels) cause the diabetic to feel some if not all of the following: thirst, increased need to pee, drowsiness, lethargy, *ickiness*, and nausea in exteme cases. Sometimes our blood sugar levels can be soaring but yet we can feel perfectly fine (John Keeler).

Hypoglycaemia   A deficiency of glucose in the bloodstream (*The Concise Oxford Dictionary*, 9th edn).

When we have too much insulin injected into our systems (also known as *insulin shock* in the USA), hypos (lows) cause the diabetic to feel some if not all of the following: dizziness, hunger, panic, fear, confusion, cold sweats, increased temperature, trembling and shaking, double vision and inability to focus or to follow instruction. Hypos, however, can vary, and some are not felt as strongly as others (John Keeler).

Insulin   A hormone produced in the pancreas by the *Islets of Langerhans* which regulates the amount of sugar (glucose) in the blood. Lack of insulin causes *diabetes* (*The Concise Oxford Dictionary*, 9th edn).

The stuff we diabetics have to inject into our bodies to try to keep our blood sugar level from rising, as we do not produce any ourselves. The insulin we inject is synthetic and is manufactured by medical companies. There are many different types of insulins on the market. I have made reference to *Actrapid*, *Monotard*, *Ultratard*, *Mixtard*, *Humalog* and *Humulin I*. Too much insulin can lead to a hypoglycaemic attack (hypo or low) and not enough may lead to hyperglycaemia (raised blood sugar) (John Keeler).

Monotard   A long-acting insulin. Injected to give the diabetic person a 'background' insulin for when the quick-acting insulin runs out. Usually lasts about 8–10 hours (John Keeler).

Ultratard A very slow-acting insulin. Injected at night to
provide background insulin being present. Reputed to
have been able to last from 24 to 36 hours in a diabetic
(John Keeler).

Index